THE ILLUSTRATED BOOK OF PHALLUSES

AF841129

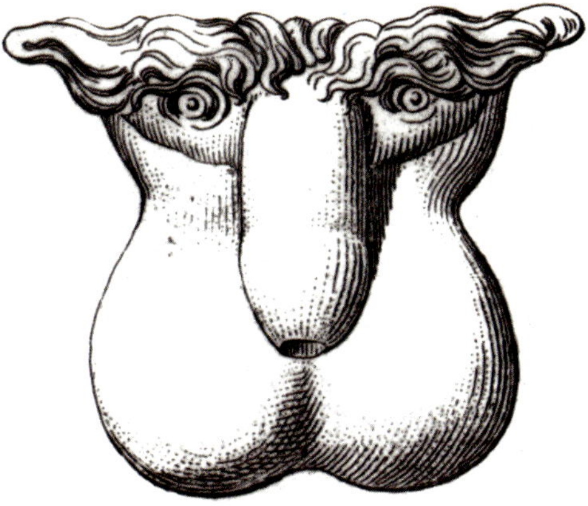

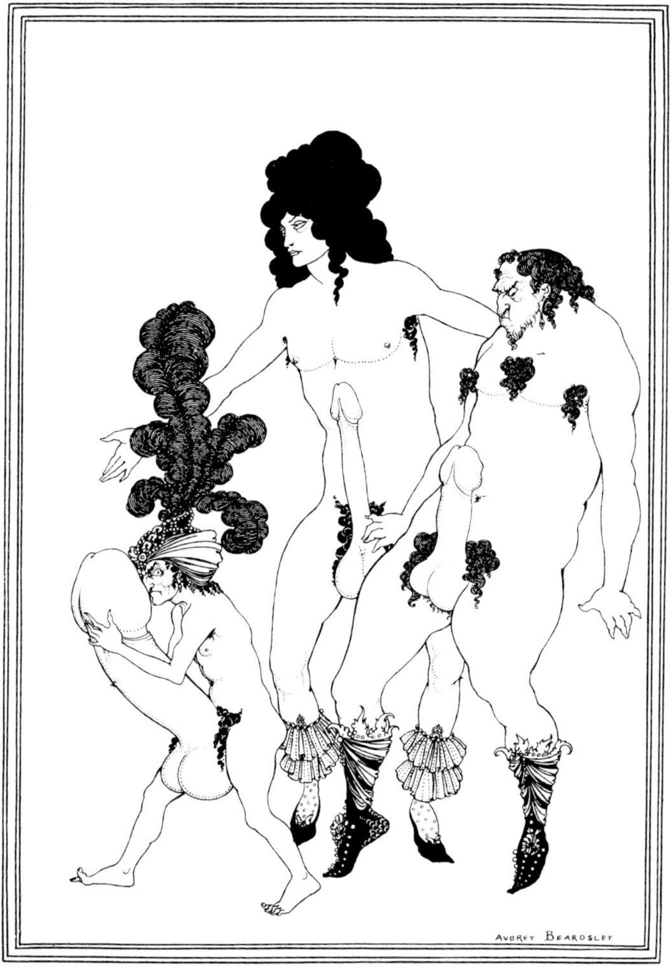
AVBREY BEARDSLEY

THE ILLUSTRATED BOOK OF PHALLUSES

A DISCURSIVE HISTORY OF THE MEMBRUM VIRILE

by

Charlotte Ward

LONDON:
THE *Erotic* Print Society
1999

ACKNOWLEDGMENTS

*The author would like to thank
the following for their help
in preparing this volume:*

*David Colvin;
Oliver Maitland; Iris Neve;
Christopher Peachment;
Christopher Routh; Mike Schofield;
James Silk; Doobie & Vikki Turney.*

Cover: Thomas Rowlandson, English (1756–1827).
The Fort.

Frontispiece: Aubrey Beardsley, English (1872–1897).
The Ambassadors.

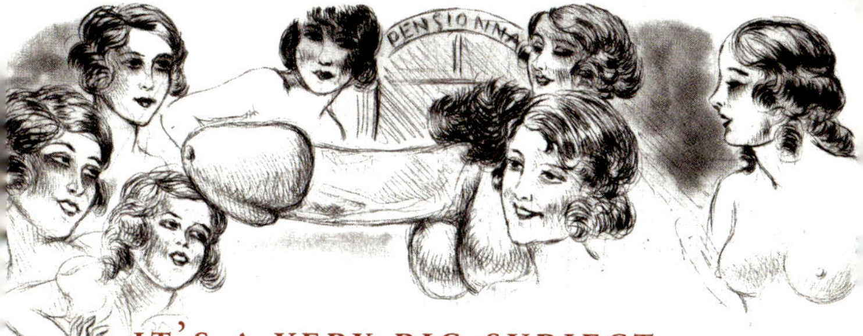

IT'S A VERY BIG SUBJECT

WHERE does one begin? In every respect, the subject is huge. It has been worshiped and revered from the beginning of time as the giver of life and joy. Only the most ardent, hard-core feminists see no beauty or worth in the penis, and portray it as a threat or weapon to be used against them and an enemy to battle with until the last drop is drained from it. They should be so lucky.

To state the obvious, where would they be without it? The todger embodies what is surely the most powerful of paradoxes. Even his detractors owe him their lives. No question about it: todgers rule.

OUR HERO EMERGES

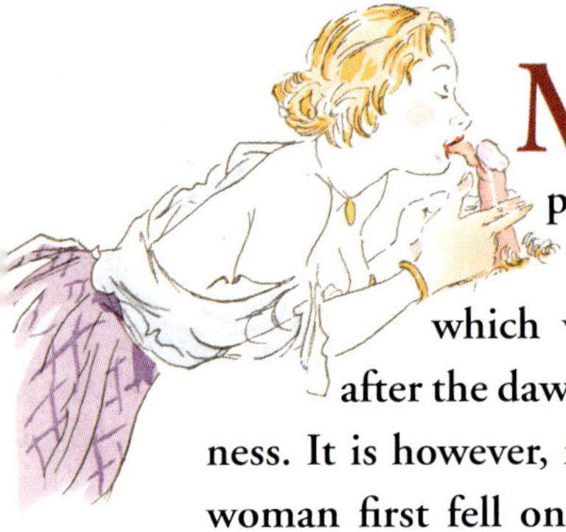

MAN has been fascinated with his penis since he first realised he had one, which was about one second after the dawn of modern consciousness. It is however, impossible to say when woman first fell on her knees before it in praise and awe. The earliest drawings and sculptures from pre-history depict figures

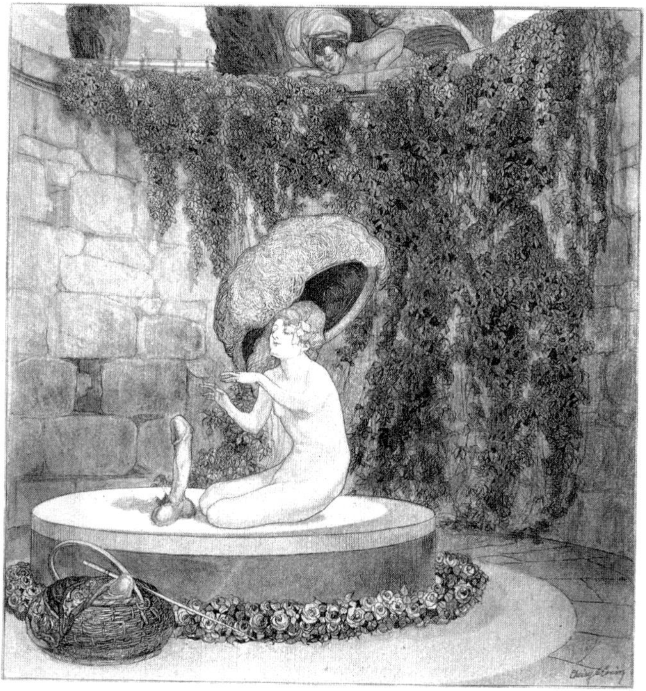

Franz, Marquis von Bayros, Austrian (1866–1924).

The Snake Charmer.

This wonderfully be-feathered lovely performs a small ritual to raise a phallus for her pleasure. She's got more waiting in the basket.

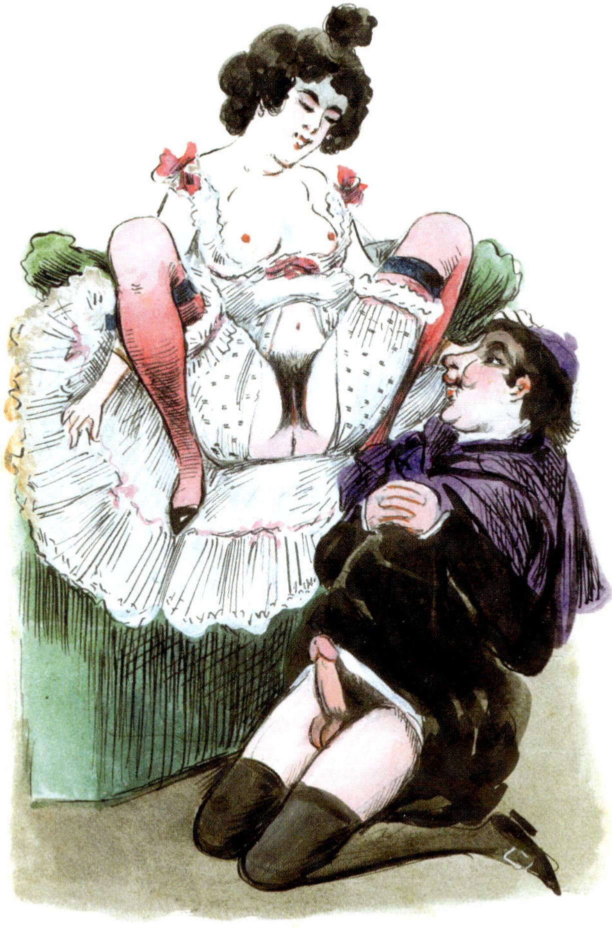

with enormous genitals, usually in the process of slaying a beast. So it would appear that the phallus was associated with power and success from the very start of recorded time. This connection is with us to this day, although now in the form of that modern black stallion, the man and his car.

In an era when little else could be relied upon, man began a love affair with his God-given pleasure stick. It served to keep him and his woman warm in winter; it didn't use up too much precious energy; he didn't have to barter to use it; and it felt great. No surprise then that our hero made an early appearance in all our mythologies.

The Cerne Giant dominates the Dorset

Unknown Artist, French (ca.1890).

A Bishop Worships at a Profane Altar.

For once this Bishop has nothing to say to the Actress. He lets his rampant crozier do the talking.

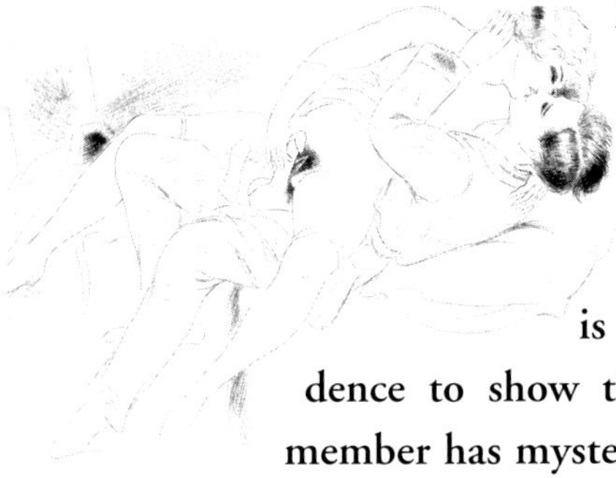

landscape like a horny Colossus, radiating fertility across the verdant countryside. There is photographic evidence to show that his remarkable member has mysteriously grown since its first documentation. Could this noble benefactor be magically extending his rich antennae in an attempt to keep apace with the population increase that we are experiencing? Experts are naturally baffled as to the cause – as with so many quasi-religious relics from our animistic past, supernatural forces conspire to mystify and confound modern rational man.

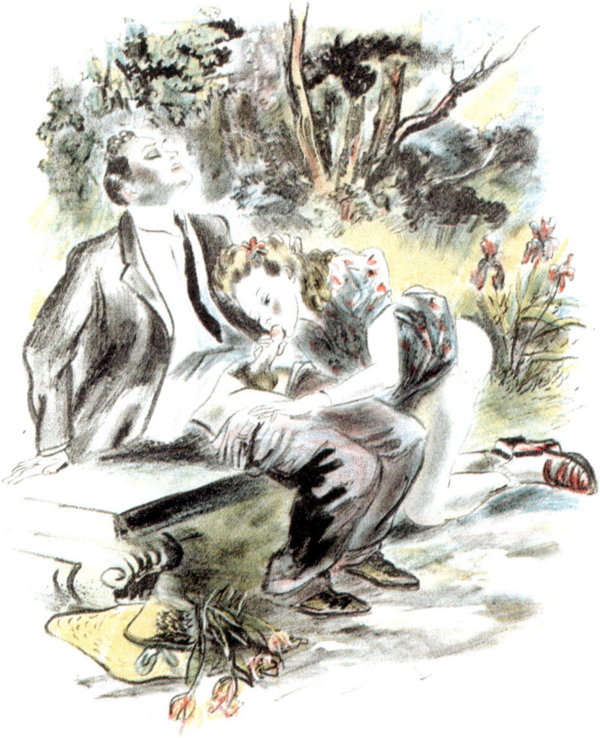

Louis André Berthommé-Saint-André, French (1905–77).

Illustration from Verlaine's *Œuvres Libres.*

It's amazing the effect a small bunch of tulips will have on an impressionable girl: the bounder has obviously picked them from the park's flowerbeds only minutes before. Lazy plucker!

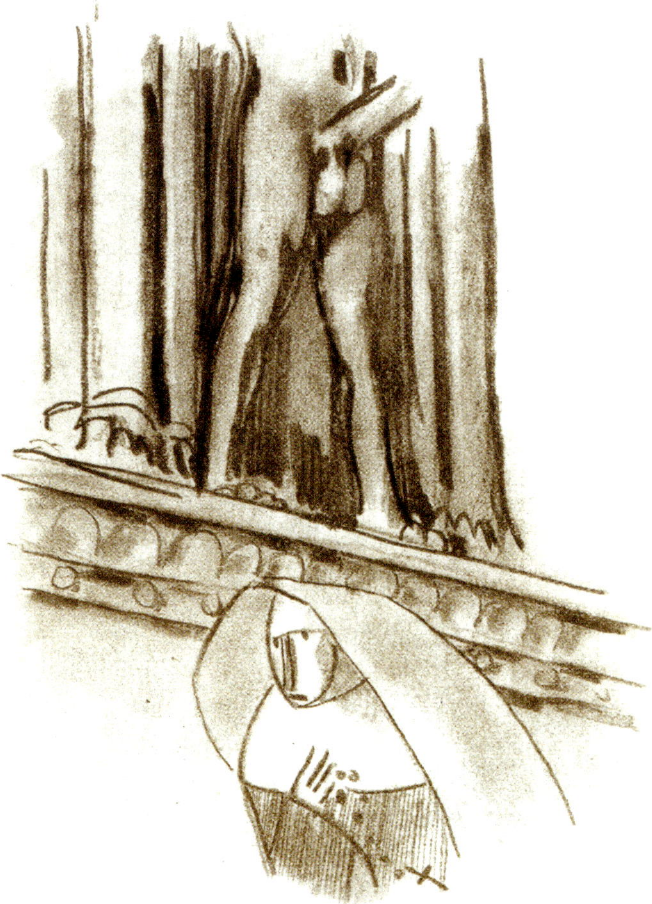

What better example of phallic worship could one find than the totem pole? One must acknowledge what a daunting prospect it is, in this post-Freudian era, to analyse objects that lend themselves so heartily to the status of phallic symbol. For as Freud himself admitted, we must remember that sometimes a cigar is just a cigar.

Let us try then to look at this pole with an impartial eye. It was originally a means of identifying tribes; by carving onto it an iconography that depicted the tribe's ancestry, the tribe could then avoid the tabu of incest. Simply stated, it dictated with whom an individual was allowed to have sexual relations. It was also believed

---

Anon., French School (ca.1930).

Illustration from *Confidences de Célestine.*

We can only sympathise with the poor mother superior's discomfiture. Her overwrought piety has magnified an innocent statue into a Priapos.

---

to possess the souls of past tribesmen, and functioned as a conduit for them to advise the tribe. On a purely realistic level however, the totem pole was a great towering structure in the centre of the reservation, which all honoured, feared and worshipped. If so respected, it would ward off evil. So if you played your cards right, you could get lucky.

Sound familiar?

Our equivalent in this country is the maypole. Our attitude towards this pole may be rather more light-hearted than that of the Native North Americans, but it is still a focal object for the community.

Anon., French (ca.1830).

Illustration from *La Pucelle d'Orléans.*

What looks like a scene from a Turkish bath. Clearly the rising herbal vapours have invigorated the young swain, not to mention a rollocking good fingering from his charming coy mistress.

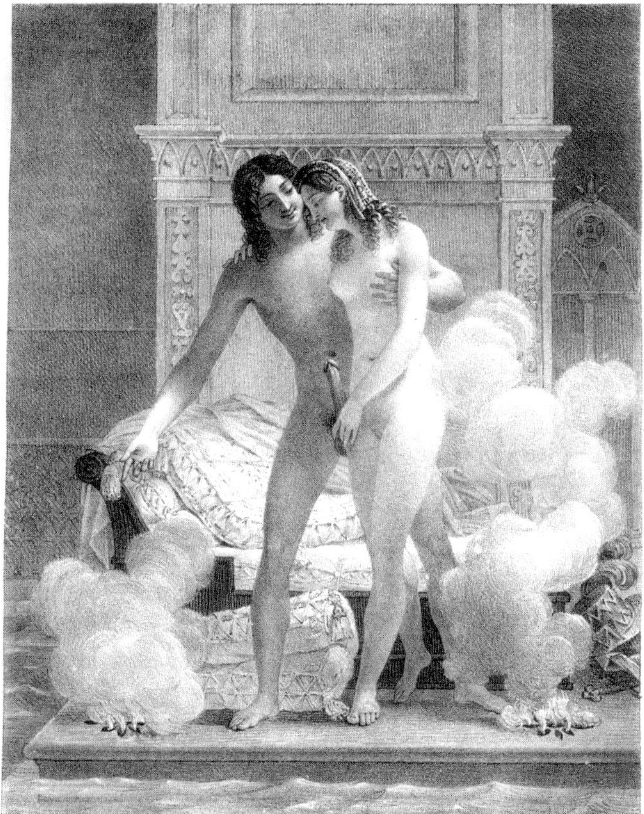

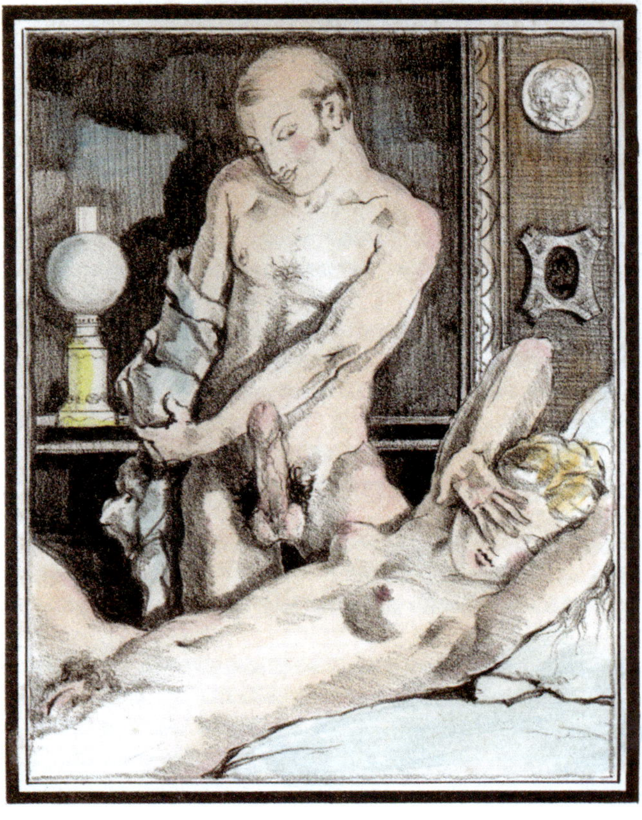

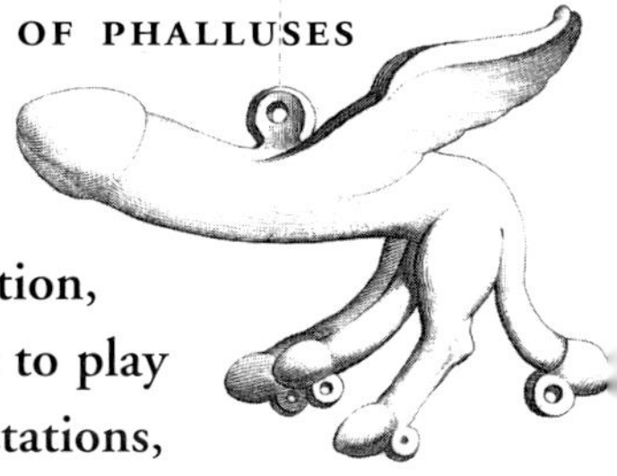

Since we are known across the globe for certain perversions involving constriction, the British feel they ought to play up to other people's expectations, and so they dance around the maypole, wrapping it all the while in tight little ribbons which slowly spiral down the full length of the shaft.

Could this have been our first communal effort at bondage, which we attempted to camouflage, centuries ago, by pretending it was a pastoral gathering that the whole family can enjoy?

Jean d'Angers, French (ca.1930).

Illustration from *Un Été à la Campagne.*

The young lady shies away in feigned horror, at the sight of his monstrous organ. She doth protest too much. Her pink upright nipples and parted nether lips betray her true feelings.

WE ANTHROPOMORPHISE HIM

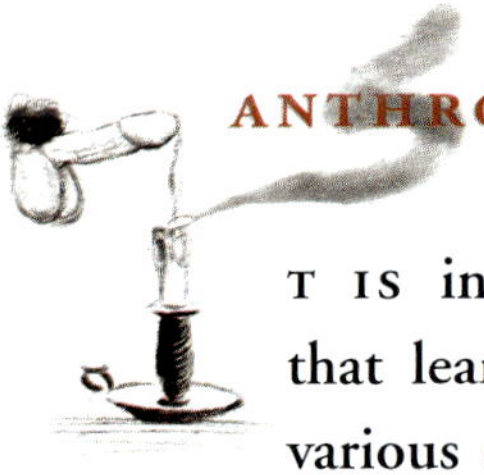

IT IS interesting to note, in a being that leans towards worship, that the various names given to the penis can also be applied to its owner: prick, dick, knob, cock-sucker etc. This is certainly not the case for the slang names of female genitalia. I can only think of one, and it is invariably applied to a man.

By the same token, it is quite common for men to talk about their members as though they were human: "He hasn't been performing well recently", is a comment frequently heard, or so my girlfriends tell me.

Anon., French (1940s).

Au Bal. Illustration from Pierre Louÿs's *Manuel de Civilité.*

This sweet-faced soubrette is clearly so proud of her young man's love machine that she just has to show it off to all and sundry. All and sundry look a mite surprised.

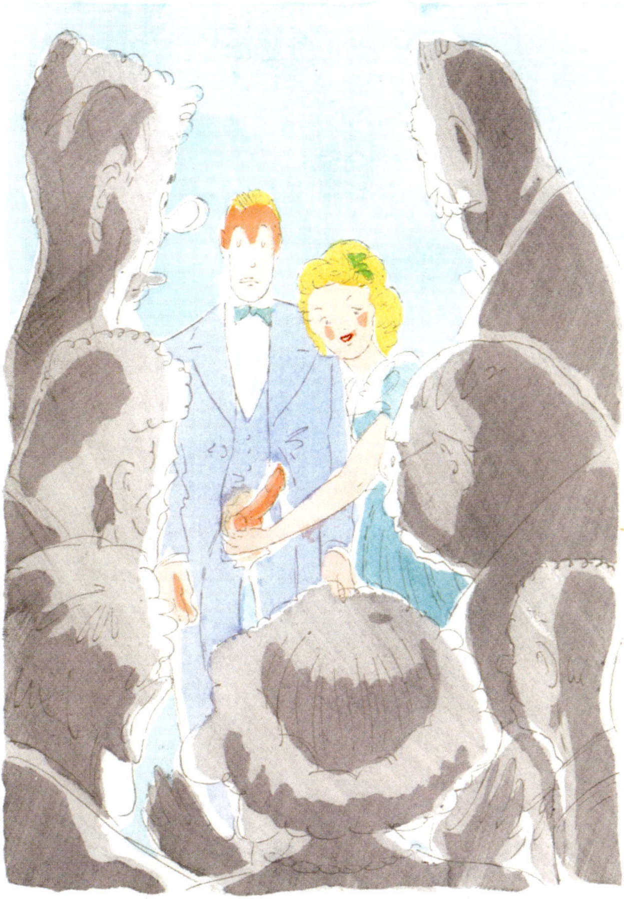

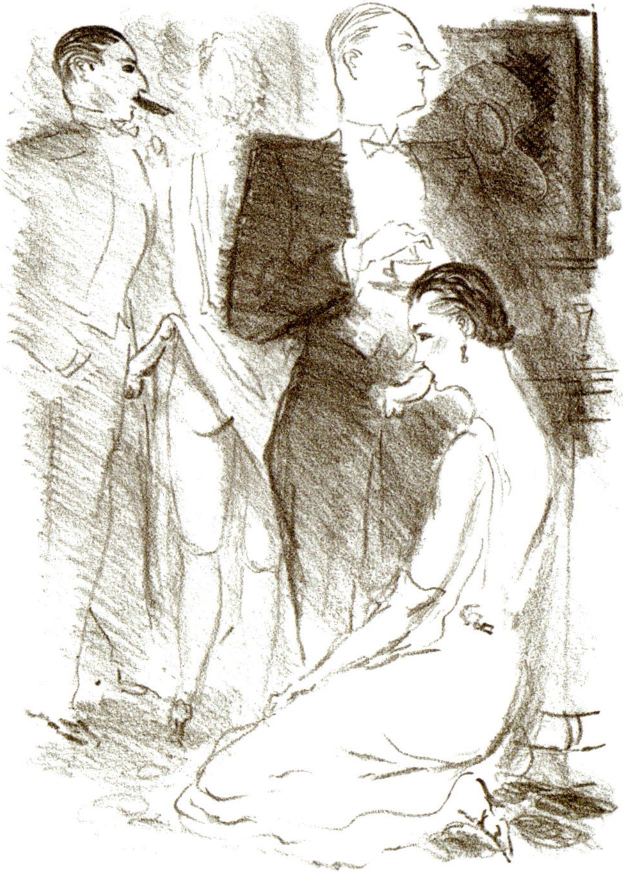

I have yet hear of a woman speaking in the same anthropomorphic fashion: "Oh she just adores a good rogering. You know me, I'm fairly casual about it, but her down there: non-stop if she could." Could this be because man has less control over his phallus, which is so prone to upsetting polite dinner parties by rearing its eager head as the hostess leans over to refill a glass and sneaking a brief glimpse into her soft cleavage? It certainly seems to lead a life of its own.

Or does this tendency of man to personify his most precious organ simply stem from the fact that it is external and

---

Marcel Vertès, Hungarian (1895–1961).

Illustration from Pierre Louÿs's *Poesies Erotiques* .

The gents in full evening fig adopt a suitable pose of *nil admirare*, in spite of the ministrations of the lightly-clad, bob-haired gels. The member in the background looks like a handy peg to hang your skirt on.

his arousal stands out so much more obviously than a woman's? If it is out, then it may as well be proud.

Either way, he is clearly a head-strong hunter, hell-bent on his *mission d'amour.*

WE ADAPT HIM

As with so many other matters concerning the todger, circumcision is a contentious issue. For many it

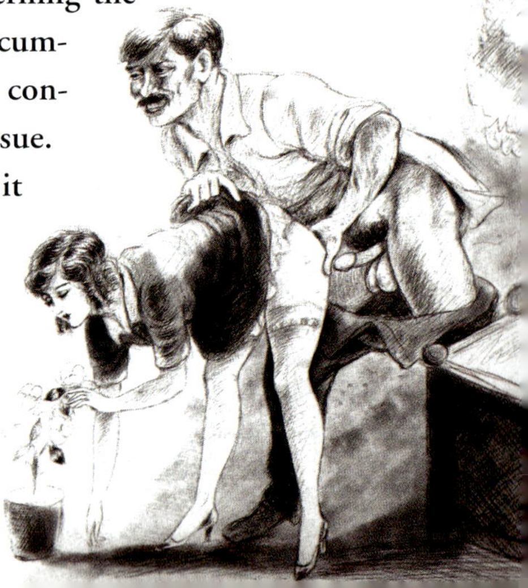

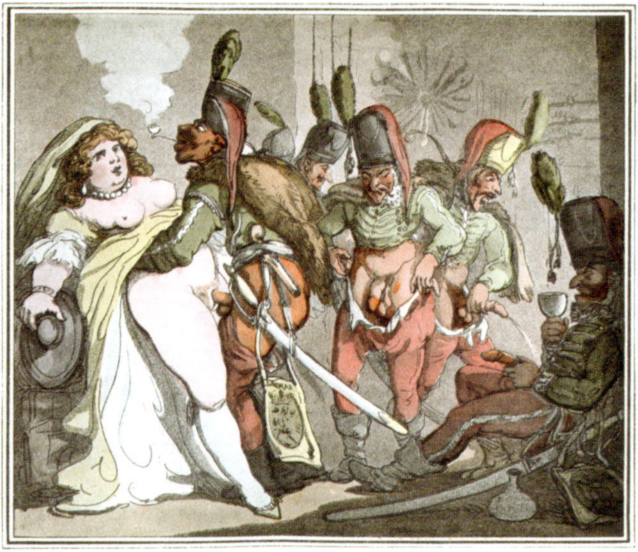

Left: Léon Courbouleix, French (active 1930s).

Illustration from *Suzon en Vacances.*

The delectable Suzon tries her hand at a little flower arranging. The gardener is about to teach her his own lesson in biological awareness.

Above: Thomas Rowlandson, English (1756–1827).

The Empress of Russia Receiving her Brave Guards.

A plump Catherine the Great gets gang-banged on a cannon by the brutal and licentious Imperial Guard. Well, what else was her Army *for*?

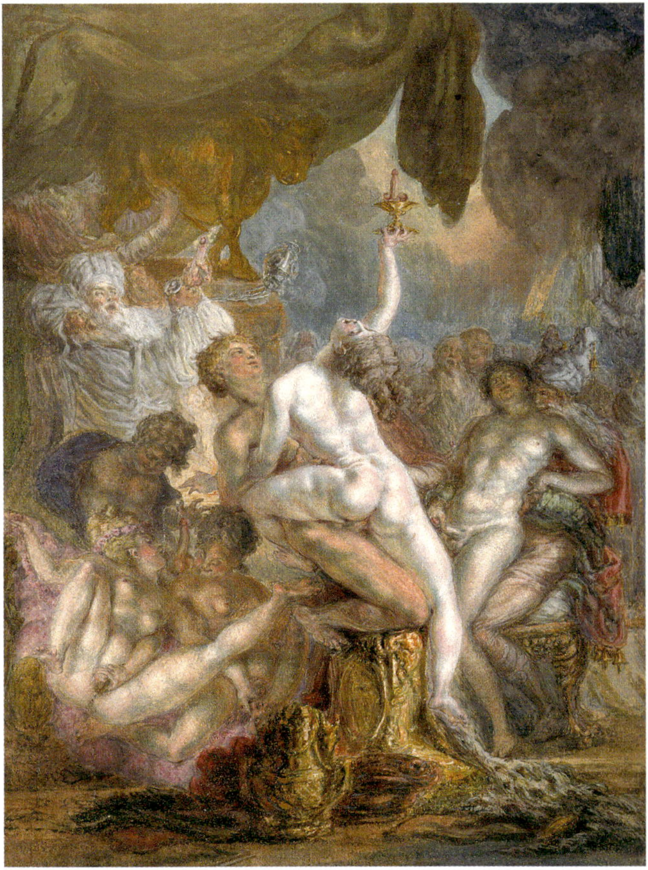

is a religious doctrine, and part of a covenant with God; others believe that it is just plain hygienic; while others view it as genital mutilation. Whatever your opinion, the operation looks as though it is not about to die out.

Jesus, following the sacred Judaic practice, is reputed to have been circumcised on 1 January. I find it interesting to note that it is one of the few aspects of Jesus's life that Christians do not insist on emulating. That, and death by crucifixion.

The Bible is quite specific on the point however:

Unknown artist, French School (ca.1750).

Adoration of the Golden Calf.

All manner of unseemly pagan delights are about to be curtailed by the appearance of Moses bearing written instructions from *Jahweh* in tablet form. "The good news is: I got Him down to ten. The bad news: Adultery is still in there."

> "And the uncircumcised man child whose flesh of his foreskin is not circumcised, that soul shall be cut off from his people." (*Genesis 17.10.*)

On the eighth day the Rabbi would perform this sacred ritual; he had a specially sharpened fingernail with which to whip it off. God seems to have been an unreasonable chap in this scenario, always expecting some form of bloody sacrifice. But then He might just have been a convenient scapegoat for men's masochism. If men really wanted to go around chopping off bits of themselves, they could at least have been honest about it and admit they did it for kicks.

Attrib. Antoine Borel, French (18th century).

Illustration from de Latouche's *Le Portier des Chartreux.*

This monastic scribe is well set up, with his special inkwell, and his even more special human lectern. Whatever he is noting down seems to be blessed with an angelic imprimatur.

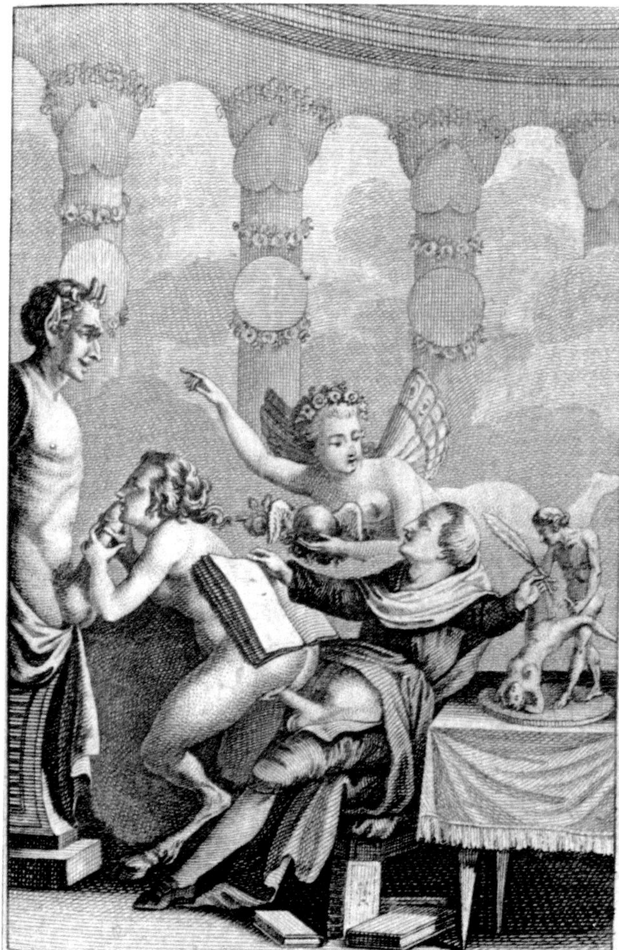

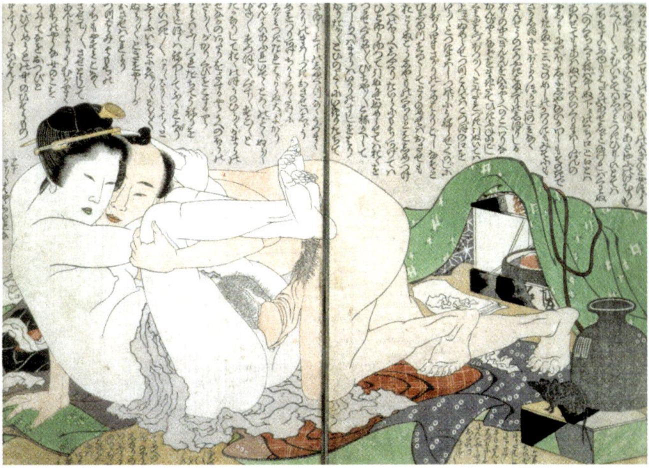

Hokusai, Japanese (1760–1849).

The Fat-bellied God of Profit.

This green-lipped beauty raises her knees for easier access. Her name is Ocase, which translates as "Let me do it".

There is some scientific evidence to suggest that circumcised men have a lower risk of penile cancer, and that the partners of circumcised men have less risk of cervical cancer. So is the foreskin a bag of nasty germs on your knob, or is there a point to it?

Tuppy Owens, a great campaigner in favour of the foreskin, went so far as to launch a magazine entitled *Foreskins Monthly.* (Personally, I prefer it more regularly.) She maintains that that little piece of skin is an essential item, and that every man should have one, for every woman to enjoy.

Doctor David Delvin, the author of *Love*

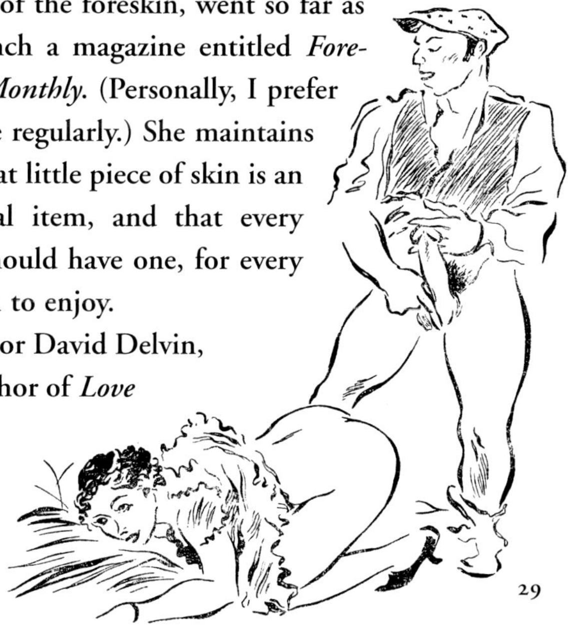

Play, describes many foreplay techniques involving the foreskin. One suggestion is to pull it fully over the head of the flaccid penis, fill it with your favourite Häagen Dazs, and slowly eat your treat. There is great joy to be had by all involved, he says.

On the other side of the debate, the circumcised man is a more enduring lover. This is due to a reduced sensitivity, caused presumably by the constantly exposed head chaffing against his flannel undies.

Pagan man, eternally looking for more extreme rituals to placate his bloodthirsty gods, didn't always stop at circumcision. No; his gods wanted the lot.

Qajar School (ca.1870).

The Pulley.

In a far pavilion, on a thick Persian carpet, a heavy-browed houri is lowered on a rope by an obliging off-stage assistant while her paramour eagerly awaits paradise. The maid looks on approvingly.

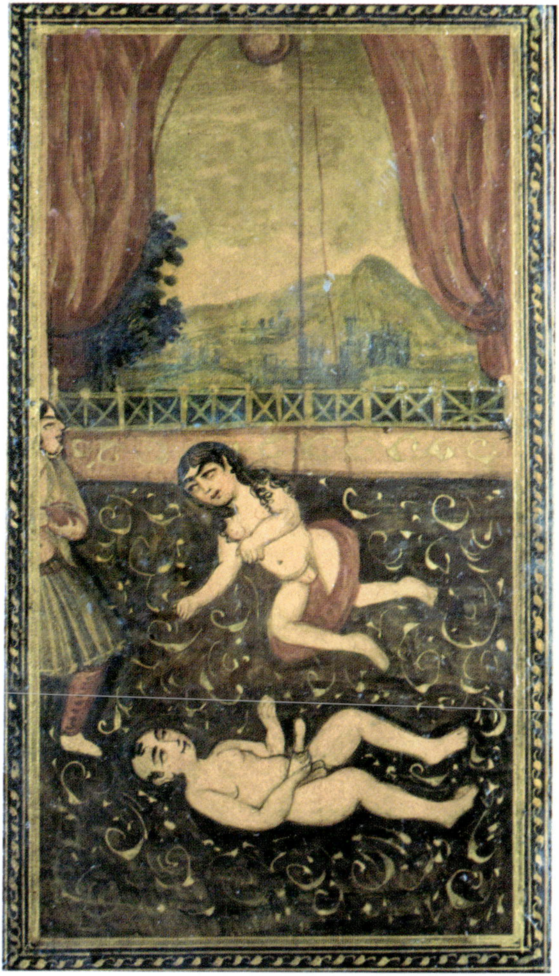

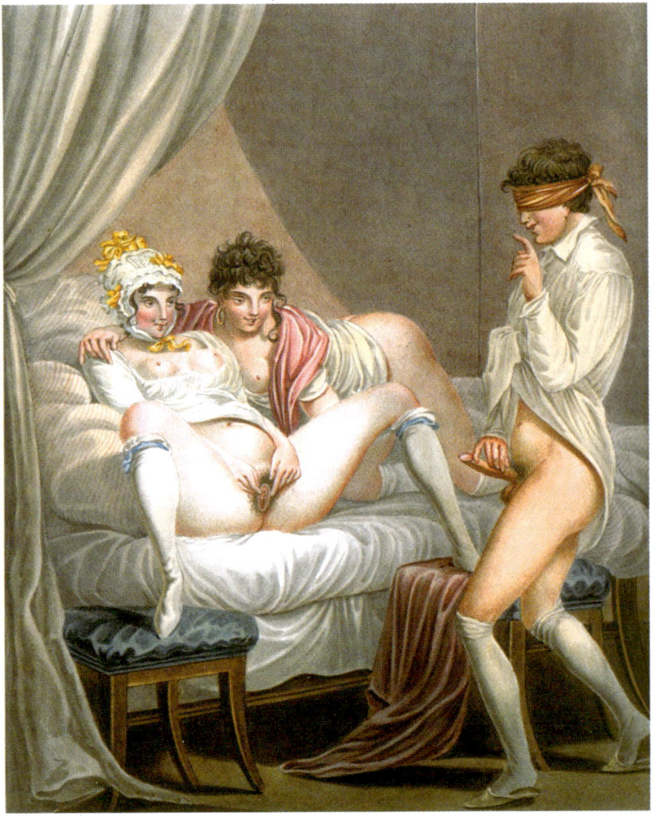

Sir James Frazer, in the *Golden Bough*, describes a street party at Hierapolis, in the Springtime:

> While the flutes played, the drums beat, and the eunuch priests slashed themselves with knives, the religious excitement spread like a wave among the crowd of onlookers, and many a one did that which he little thought to do when he came as a holiday spectator to the festival. For man after man, his veins throbbing with the music, his eyes fascinated by

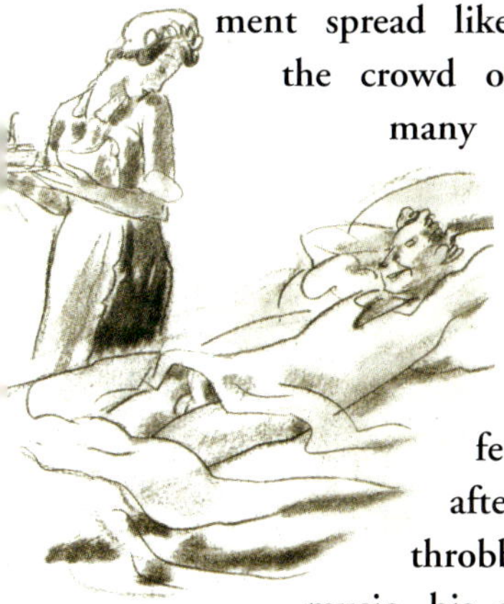

Left: Georg Emmanuel Opitz, Czech/German (1775–1841). *Blind Man's Buff.*

A lady in a jaunty Jane Austen tea-cosy hat eagerly awaits her just prize in this lewd variation on the traditional parlour game. Her friend sportingly offers no competition.

> the sight of the streaming blood, flung his garments from him, leaped forth with a shout, and seizing one of the swords which stood ready for the purpose, castrated himself on the spot.

The modern reader may find the above practice both alarming and extreme. But then he should consider the current renaissance that body piercing is enjoying. It follows from a similar mania for self-

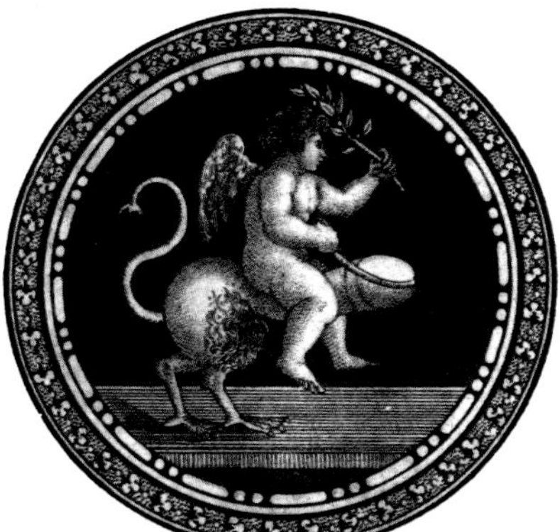

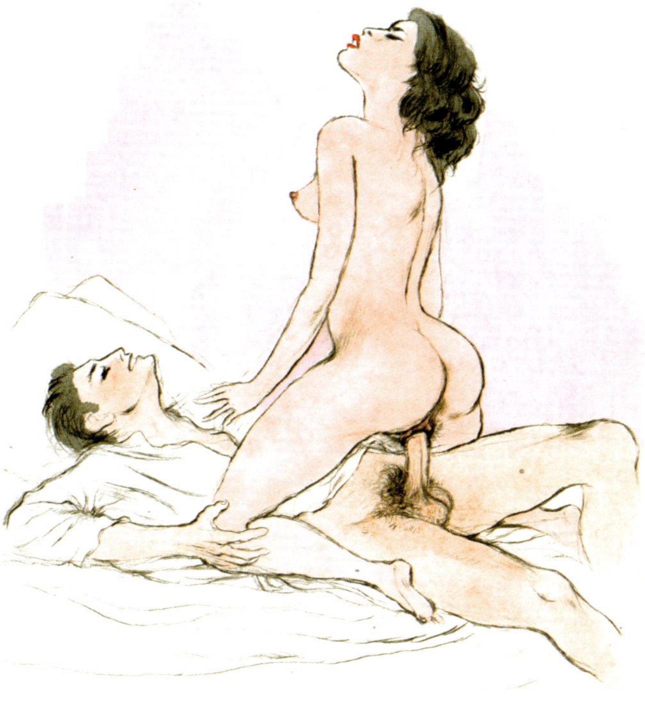

Above: Anon., French (ca.1939).

Illustration from *Séduction.*

She looks deadly serious, as well she might, since she is just about to be impaled on a mighty prong.

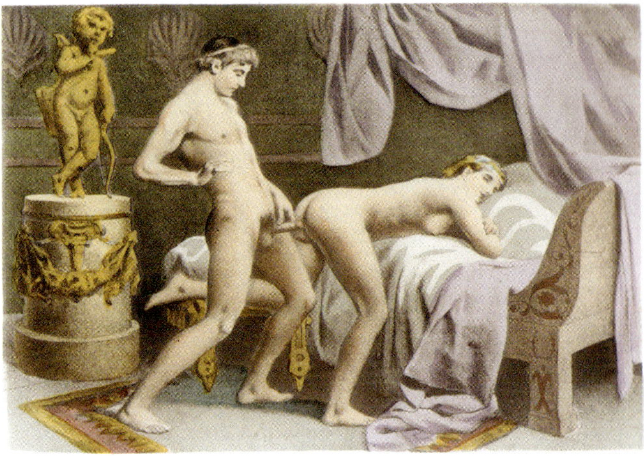

Paul Avril, French (1849–1928).

Aloisius. From *De Figuris Veneris.*

"Tunc pronus inclinat se in nates Aloisius. Pilum postico admovet, pulsat, percutit, post summo nisu irrumpit." Bad luck if you don't have a classical education, as this fragment of Chorier is really rather rude.

mutilation, even if it seldom goes as far as clean-shaven castration. Its devotees are passionate about the practice. When Billy Connolly had his nipples pierced, his assailant said: "One more of us, one less of them". It has about it something of a devotional activity, like the masochistic quests of mediæval knights. We are still in the early days of the piercing renaissance, and there may yet be much more startling uses for steel rings and studs than we have yet imagined.

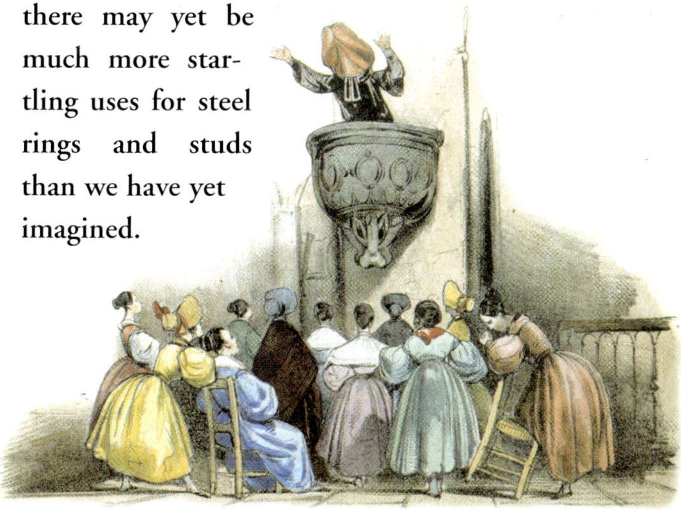

WE ADORN HIM

PENIS piercing is a fairly common practice these days, though not for the faint of heart. Having a large hoop inserted through the head is called a Prince Albert, and is one of the more extreme methods employed. This popular form of self-mutilation is not named, as the myth has it, after Queen Victoria's saintly husband, but after the wicked

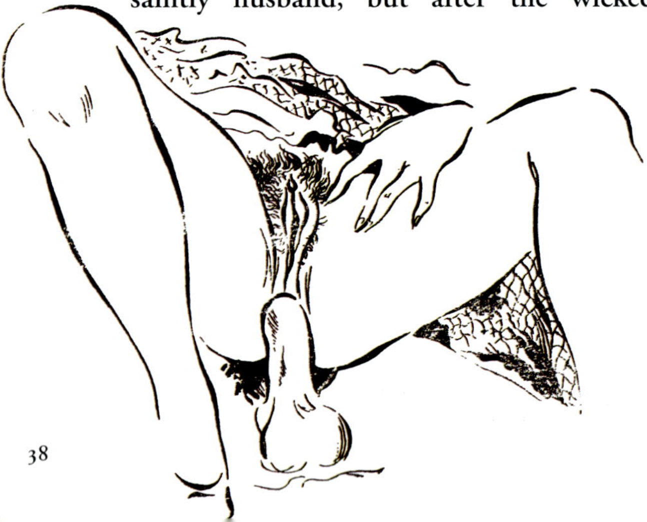

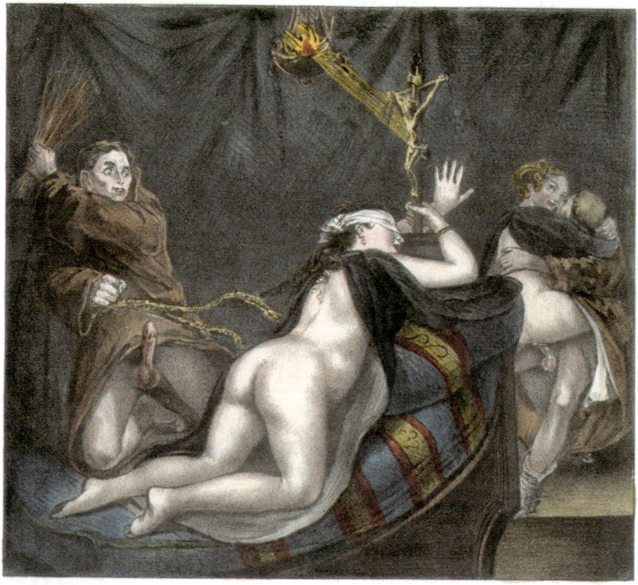

Achille Deveria, French (1800–1857).

Monastic Pleasures. Illustration from *Gamiani.*

The blindfolded, virginal Countess Gamiani has been duped by her wicked Aunt (enjoying herself in the background) into entering a monastery full of priapic monks. A fondly remembered and formative experience from her youth.

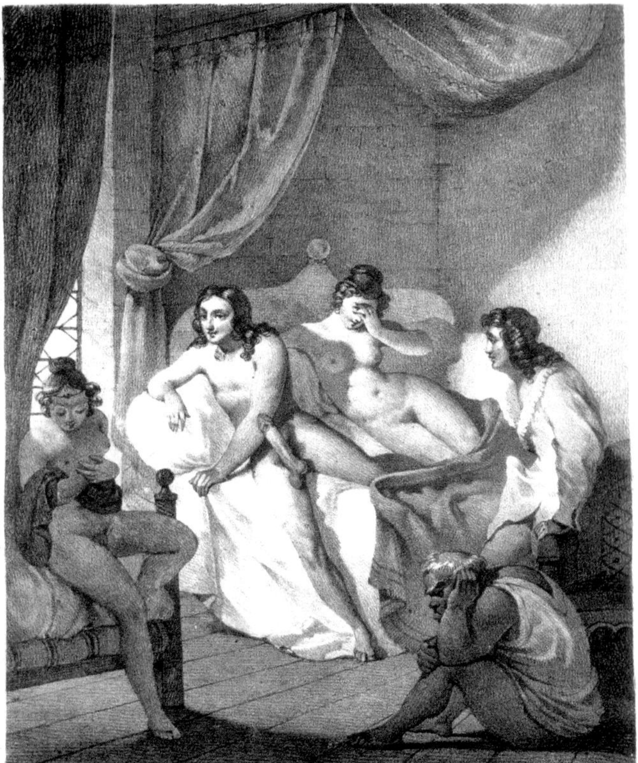

Duke of Clarence, mooted as Jack-the-Ripper, and their grandson. He was said to have had a member so prodigious that it was prone to playing up by itself, and in an attempt to control his wayward knob he would lash it to his leg with a chain. It seems a most utilitarian attitude to have to your helmet, but it reportedly made his dresser's job easier, and also helped avoid the danger so common when horse-riding in a high-pommelled saddle.

If the rumours of his sheer size were true, it does suggest greediness on his Highness's part to have indulged in even greater pleasure-giving adornments.

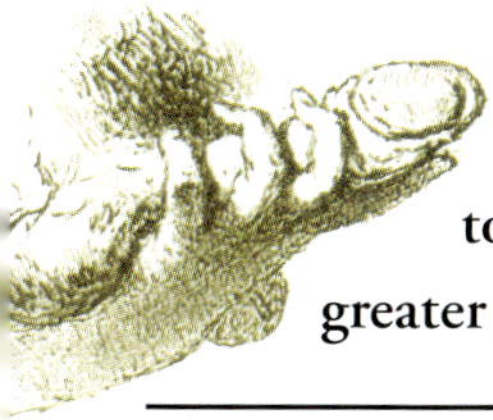

Anon., French (ca.1830).

Illustration from *La Pucelle d'Orléans.*

The blushing maidens hardly know where to look, when confronted with such a mighty organ. Although the one in the middle is sneaking a good peek through her fingers.

Who could compete? Not only did Bertie have a large battalion, but it was fully armed.

Weights can also be attached to the Prince Albert to strengthen and lengthen the penis. It is uncertain whether strengthening is actually achievable or even beneficial – except for party tricks. There is always one prick standing at the door holding coats on his knob – if you go to the right parties that is. In some African tribes, however, it seems that the lengthening is so heartily pursued that it is necessary to tie a knot in the middle of the member. This may be attractive to

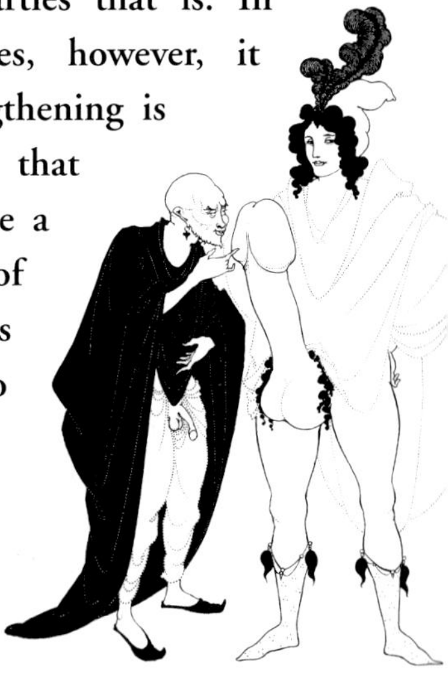

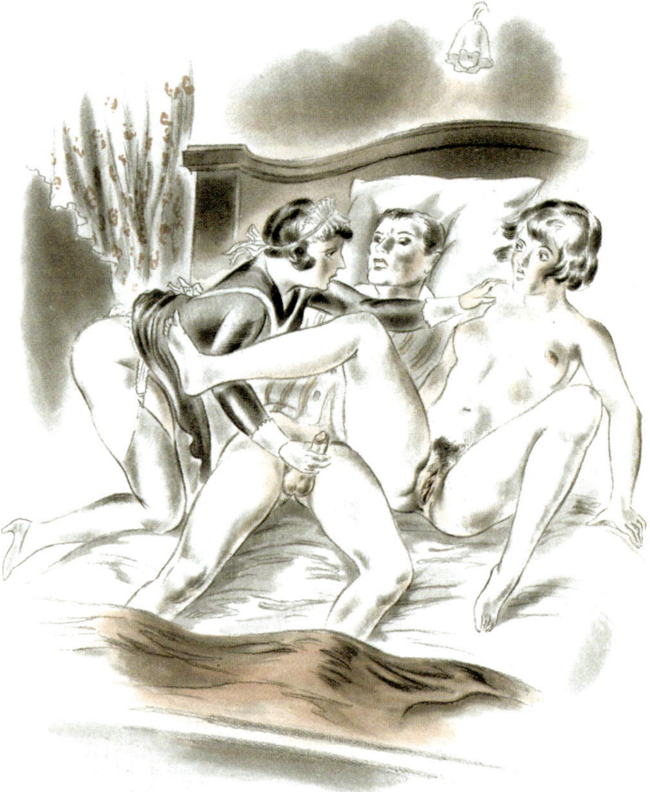

Louis André Berthommé-Saint-André, French (1905–77).

La Femme de Chambre. From *Pybrac.*

Everybody ought to have a maid. Especially for increasing the ardour of a jaded marriage bed. This maid is angrily displacing the lady of the house. "It's my turn," she cries.

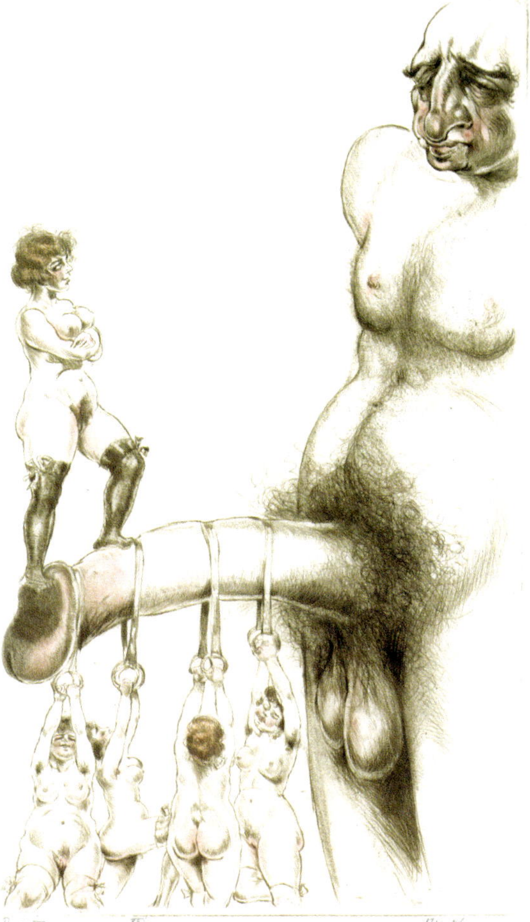

some, but strikes me as not just cumbersome but fantastically unnecessary.

The famously well-endowed porn star King Dong is famously unable to enjoy a full erection without passing out. His member requires so much blood that his brain becomes starved. What, then, is the point of having all that love but be unable to stay conscious for long enough to use it? It is surely a complete and flagrant waste of flesh. The point about a todger is surely that its appeal is not purely aesthetic. Far better to have a cosily accommodated and useful cock.

So far as piercing goes, the Kama Sutra

"Pipifax", German (ca. 1920).

From *Erotische Grotesken.*

He may look a little old and mournful, but his weapon is still mighty enough to let four buxom Rhine maidens do their swing gymnastics on it. Not to mention the naked dark hussy brazenly stomping on his glans. He should be so lucky.

got there first, as with so many issues erotic. It details the Apadravya: a double headed stud, inserted through the head and urethra, and corresponding in size to his partner's Yoni. There is no male benefit to this form of piercing; it is purely to enhance the female's pleasure. The nature of the stimulation that this particular stud gives suggests that something was known of the elusive G-spot centuries ago. And further evidence that in our reluctance to improve our pleasurable pursuits we slow-witted Westerners are way behind the East.

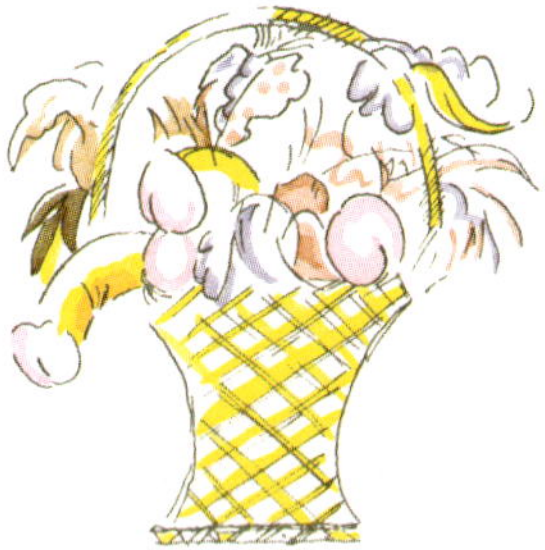

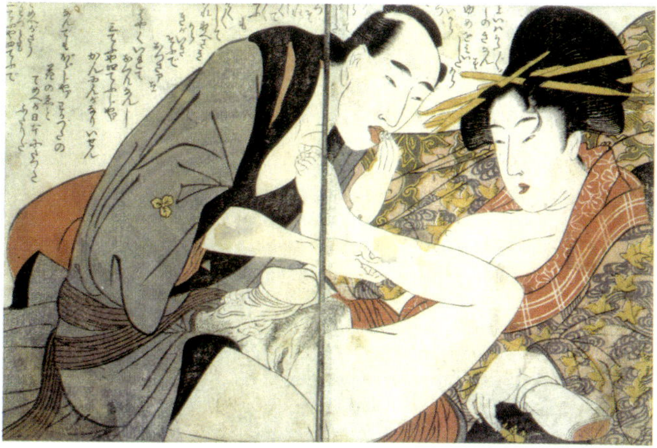

Utamaro, Japanese (1757–1806).

In the Brothels of Yedo.

The male lover licks his fingers to lubricate his mighty weapon and make entry easier, while she waits in ecstasy.

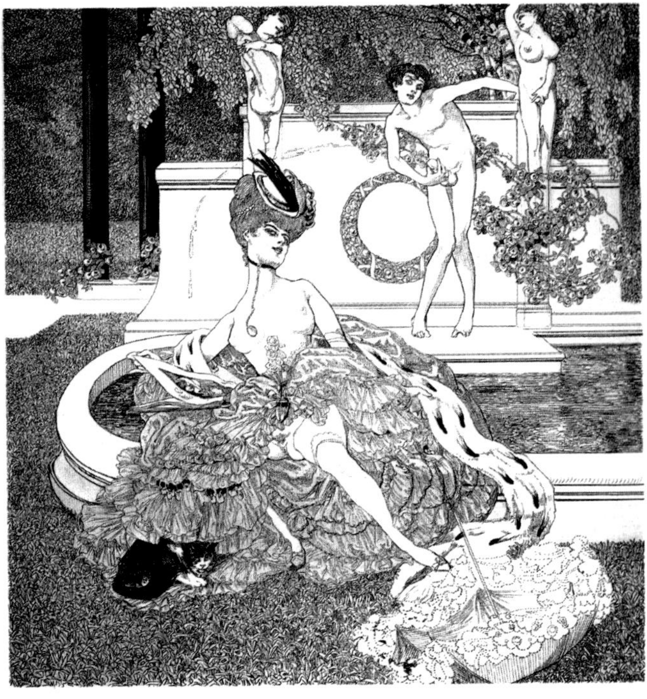

Franz, Marquis von Bayros, Austrian (1866–1924).

Der Bote.

Which means "The Ambassador". We can only suppose the good marquis is referring to the truly prodigious amount of ejaculate that is arcing its way to an unsuspecting reader.

WE GET THE MEASURE OF HIM

THERE is a common myth (never proved), that the size of the penis corresponds to the size of the hands, feet or nose. I suppose this does give those of us with ape-like appendages something of a chance in today's dating arena, dominated as it is by elfin androgynes. A woman is more likely to entertain a Yeti with the nose of a manatee, if she thinks

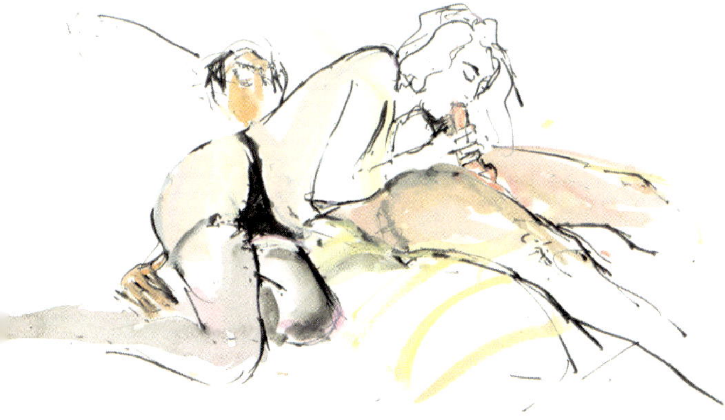

his nose is a harbinger of the python in his pants.

One girlfriend of mine told me about the antics of one of her conquests. This young chap strutted around her sitting room with his palm extended, indicating the whole palm-span from the tip of his pinkie to the top of his thumb, and assuring her that she would not be disappointed. "Cock-sure," I thought. Fortunately he wasn't lying, but apparently it was the only thing he was sure about, which leads me to ponder this possible correlation.

Just as the very beautiful do not have to trouble themselves with the effort of developing a personality, by the same token, the

---

Jean Dulac, French (active 1920–40).

Illustration from *Nous Deux*.

Hello sky! Hello clouds! This young lovely has removed her skirt the better to enjoy nature's bounteous offerings, which in this case include a large male member.

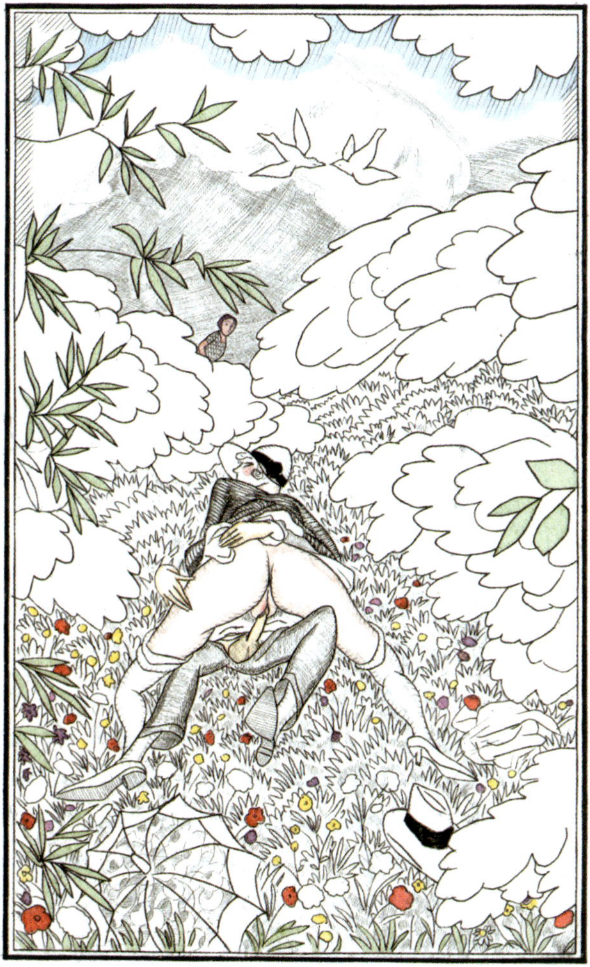

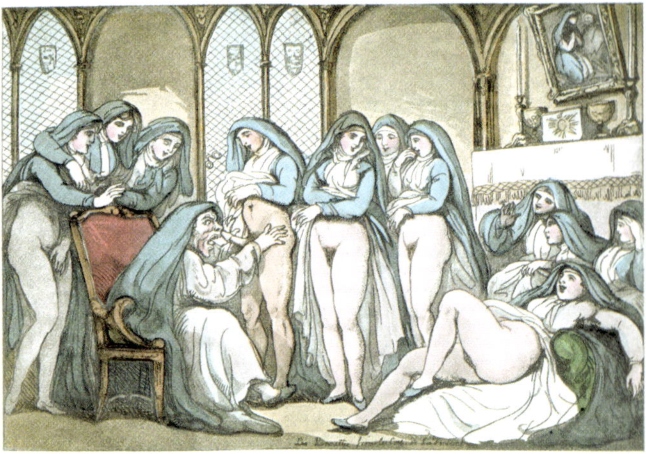

Thomas Rowlandson, English (1756–1827).

The Spectacles.

An illustration to a story of La Fontaine. No one remembers the plot but it involves an ugly Mother Superior, her spectacles, some playful nuns and a randy male gardener *en travestie.*

very well-hung can rely upon their super-rods to save them from solitude. Many women I know will suffer an intolerable berk, if he carries a Smith and Wesson down his trousers. Indeed, I too have been guilty of this superficiality of character in my own seedy past.

Many believe that there is no connection between the various body sizes at all, and it is all simply a matter of heredity. My personal belief though is that it is the thumb which provides a taste of things to come. Just as palmists read the lines on your hands, so can I read the structure of the thumb. The width and length of the digit, in relation to the rest of the hand, gives a clue to the proportion of the phallus to the owner. The

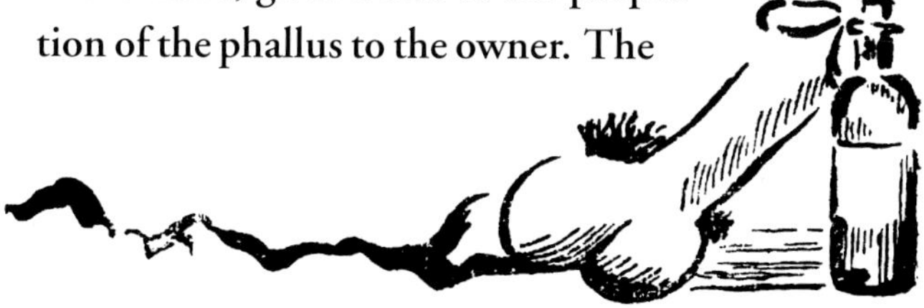

overall shape and curves, (bending forward from knuckle for example, or swelling at the same point) I have found to be replicated in the penis. It even extends to the way that the nail joins the skin, and the area it occupies, being similar to the shape and dimensions of the head or helmet. Go ahead, have a good comparative look.

As a theory it remains unproved, but I'm working hard on the research. Of course there is no way of totally avoiding that moment of delight or disappointment, when you feast your eyes for the very first time on your lover's member. And, alas, there are often shocks. I had a Danish *beau* once, who had skin the colour of vanilla fudge.

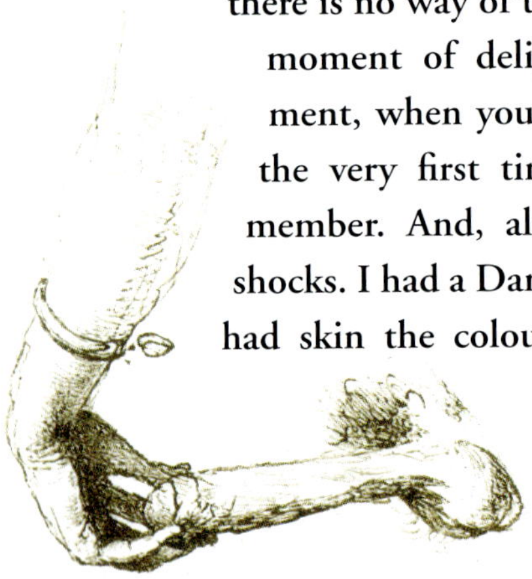

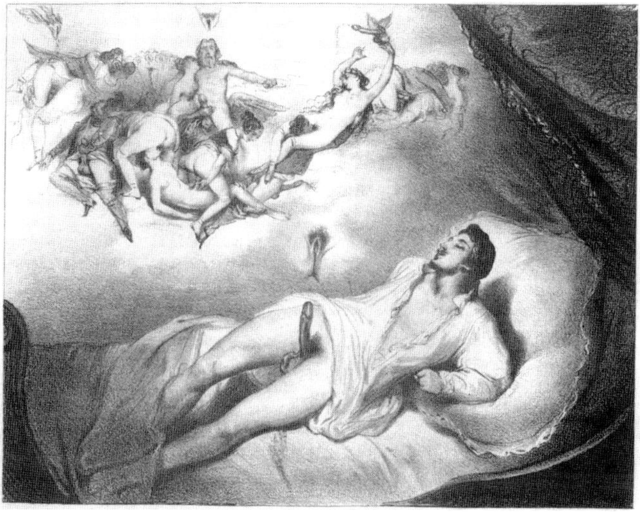

Achille Deveria, French (1800–57).

A Dream of Mount Olympus. Illustration from *Gamiani.*

An oneiric vision of Jupiter, Juno and the whole Greek host of gods on Olympus gives this happy sleeper an erection that the cat could use as a scratching post.

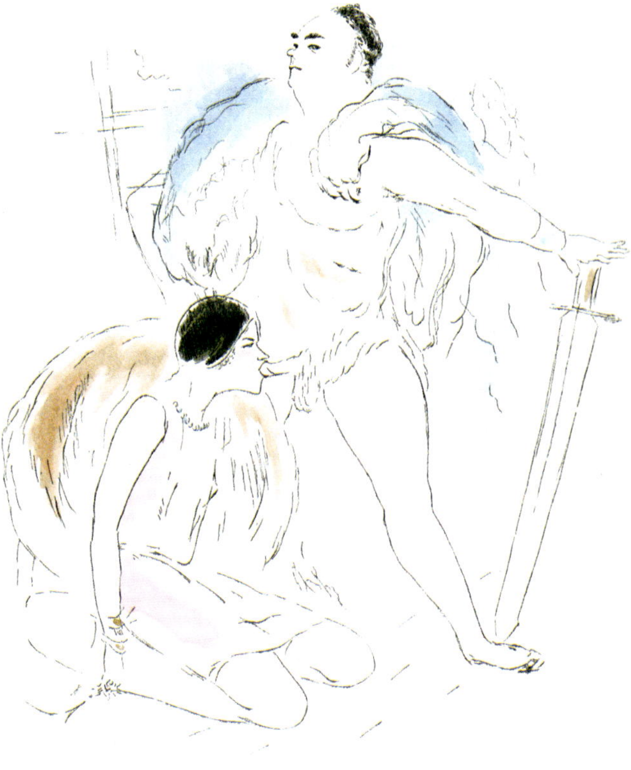

Imagine my surprise when I discovered that his entire lingam was a sooty black, and quite incongruous to the rest of his body. And in case you're wondering, no, his thumb wasn't discoloured, you can only force a theory so far. What's more, its nice not to have the territory all mapped out before you get there.

HOLISTIC HERO

USUALLY our happy little hunter confidently seeks out his prey and, rising to the occasion, goes boldly in to do

---

Marcel Vertès, Hungarian (1895–1961).

Illustration from *Pybrac.*

He might not have the face of a hero, but the bear-skins, the hefty broad sword and the mighty weapon all proclaim a modern Hercules. The lady in the fetching cloche hat knows her place in the scheme of things.

battle. However this is not always the case. Sometimes he is simply not up to the task. Most men experience impotence, at some time in their lives. The reasons for this malaise are as various as the men who are prone to it. In our modern analytical

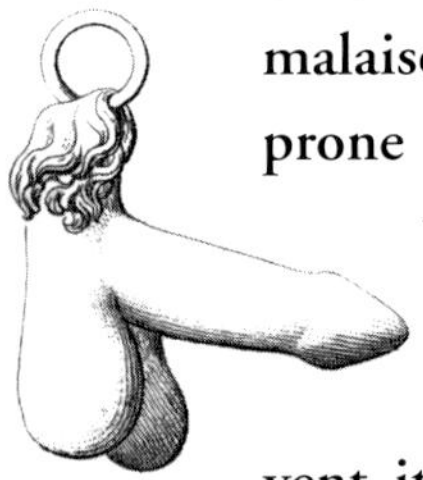

world, it is held that most cases of impotency are psychological. If this is so, what can men do to prevent it? Perhaps they should think about the problem less and find a way to avoid over-complicating the act of love.

Men are under enormous pressure these days to fulfil numerous contradictory roles, and in my opinion, the role of being a good

---

Mihaly von Zichy, Hungarian (1827–1906).

From *Liebe.*

A thoughtful early study of the delights of mouth to todger resuscitation. "Blow bugle blow. Set the wild echoes flying" as Tennyson, who looked rather like this lucky fellow, put it.

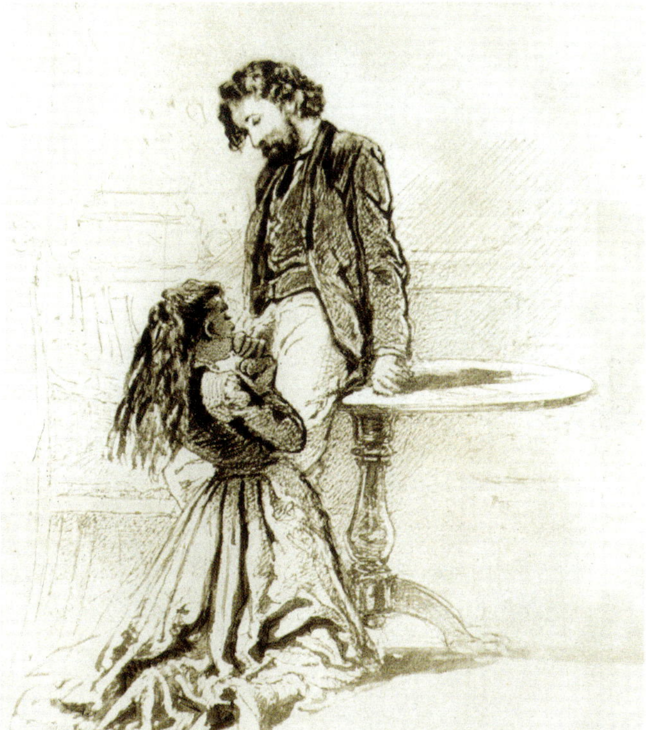

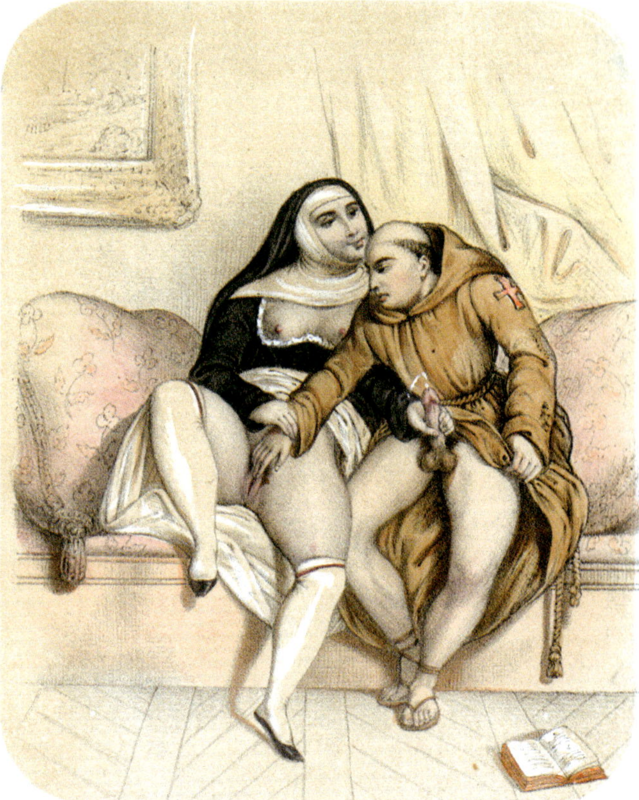

"lover" has been relegated. Many male friends of mine complain of being too tired, or stressed out by their jobs, or of family commitments. Or they may feel threatened by what they perceive as aggression from today's sexually liberated women. The possibilities are endless.

The idea of simply enjoying an evening with an attractive woman, walking her home, being invited in for coffee, and in the early hours coupling frantically like dogs on heat, more often fills them with dread than adrenaline. What if she's had better, more gymnastic, more imaginative lovers in the past? All these anxieties push the blood to the brain and away from its

French School (early 19th century).

L'Education du Jeune Novice.

Nothing like the vows of chastity to get the juices flowing. This couple are clearly neglecting their bible studies in favour of playing Adam and Eve.

intended target, leaving him limp and defeated.

My darling boys, I urge you to remember that we are on your side. No woman that I know of lies in wait for the opportunity to humiliate and ridicule the man she has taken as her lover, laughing at his inability and pointing at his inadequacy.

I say "no woman I know of", but upon reflection this is clearly untrue. I know of many. However they either have an intensely refined taste for domination or they charge a fortune.

So rest assured, we girls are not hyper-critical, whip-wielding, over-demanding, voracious sex bitches (unless you ask me very sweetly). Neither do our cunts have

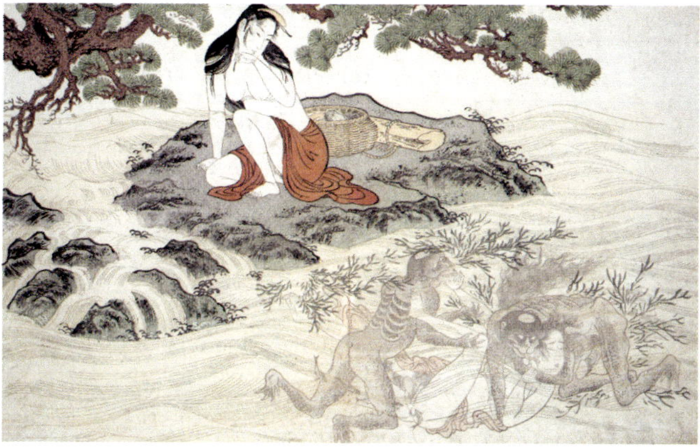

Utamaro, Japanese (1753–1806).

Kappa (*River Monsters*) *Violating a Fisher Girl.* From the *Utamakura* (*Poem of the Pillow*) 1788.

Two speckled sea beasties with webbed hands and feet, use their long tongues and longer phalli to violate an unfortunate fisher girl. Her *Awabi* diving partner looks on in dismay.

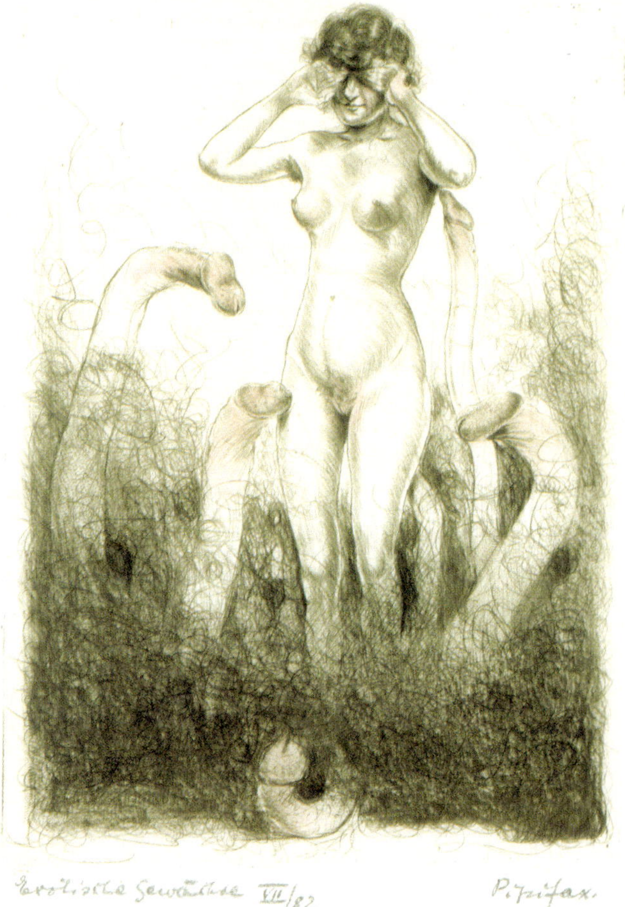
Erotische Gewächse VII/82

teeth, in order to tear your best friend off at its root and throw your parts from speeding cars (unless you're very unlucky, and have an alternative career lined up as a cockless chat show guest). We want the same as you. Wine me, dine me, sixty-nine me. Isn't that what you want too?

Once again, it is the Kama Sutra which maps out the perfect evening of seduction. It gives full details of receiving the woman in "the pleasure room", talking suggestively, singing, playing musical instruments and drinking. And all of this before any kissing or fondling takes place. When the woman is overcome with desire, the man should try to

---

"Pipifax", German (ca.1920).

From *Erotische Grotesken.*

A poor bemused young thing looks a bit put out by her dream of being set upon by a colony of rampant, one-eyed serpents.

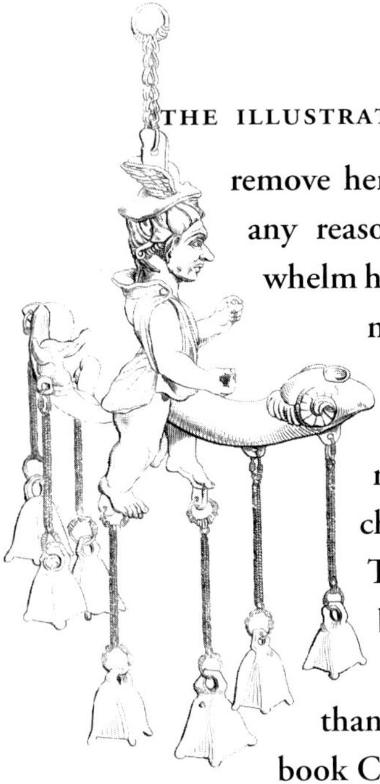

remove her clothes, "if she resists for any reason he should try to overwhelm her with kisses on her cheeks, making her breathlessly excited". It all seems so easy, and I'm sure, for many, this foolproof flowchart for seduction works. The essential ingredient is a belief in what you are doing. There is nothing worse than being seduced by a textbook Casanova, who is more interested in his own ability to bed you, than your actual arousal. A certain degree of shared interest is always polite.

Thomas Rowlandson, English (1756–1827).

The Itinerant Entertainers.

A miraculous balancing act by this well-endowed jongleur inspires the crowd to throw coins into his young assistant's gratefully upheld skirts.

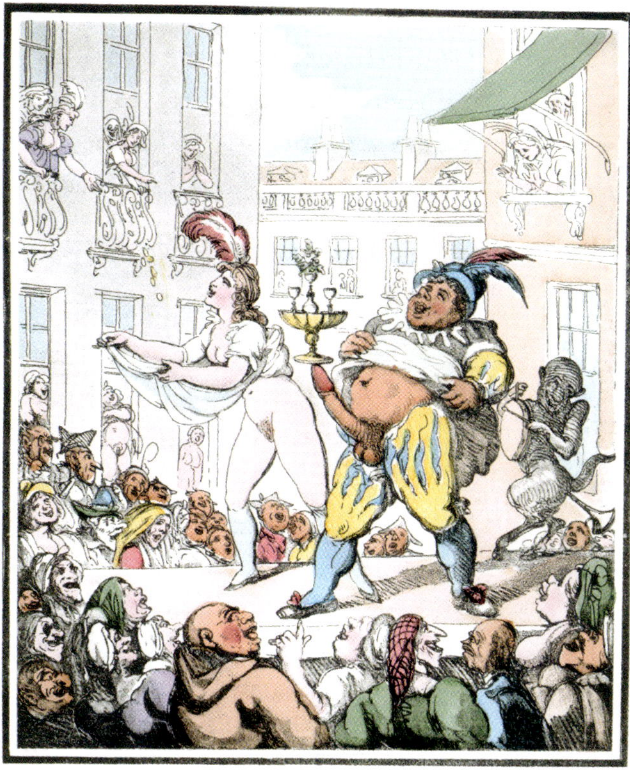

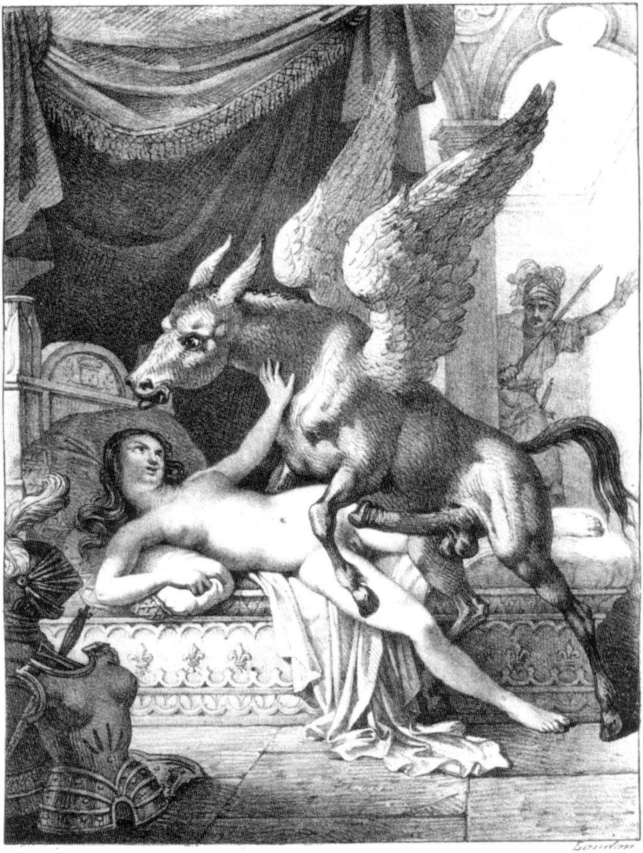

It must then come down to the man's expectations of his tool. How often should you realistically expect sex? Does your lover need a performance, or are they happy with something more subdued? If you feel your interest flagging, how can you revive the old fella?

Now, there is nothing like taking a vow of celibacy to get your blood pumping and your juices flowing. Just look at the habits of any restrictive religious order, and you will find the most rampant and debauched sexual practices. Abstinence makes your parts grow stronger. Sadly though there are just not enough monasteries to keep apace

Anon., French (ca.1830).

Illustration from *La Pucelle d'Orléans.*

Mercy! *Another* donkey. Although this one has the sensible addition of wings, the better to hover above his evening's mount. The good lady goes through the motions of refusal, but her face says otherwise. She's seen the size of him.

with the rise in impotency, and so both sexes must pull together, to try to overcome this upsetting condition.

A husband and his wife are experiencing some difficulties with their sex-life, and find discussing it embarrassing. Eventually the husband turns to his wife and says: "Now, my darling, I think I may have the answer here. As and when you do want to have sex, which is obviously fine by me, you simply reach over and gently tug my John Thomas once. When you don't want to have sex, which is equally fine, you reach over and tug it about one hundred and fifty times."

I'm rather drawn to a quaint Judaic tra-

Anon., French (1940s).

Devoirs Envers Votre Mère. Illustration to *Manuel de Civilité.*

Our strawberry-cheeked soubrette smiles so sweetly as she generously lends her young man's love machine to her mother for a good two-hander.

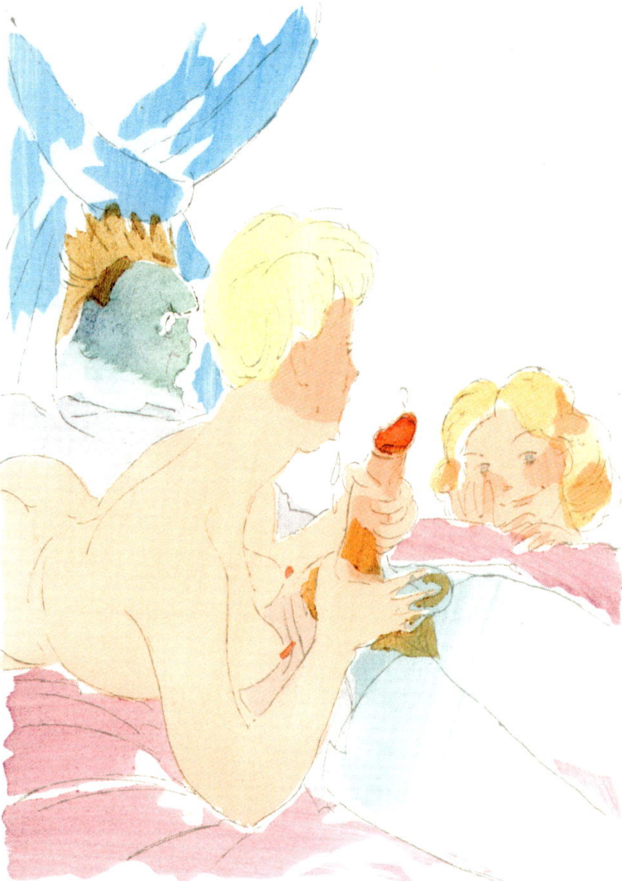

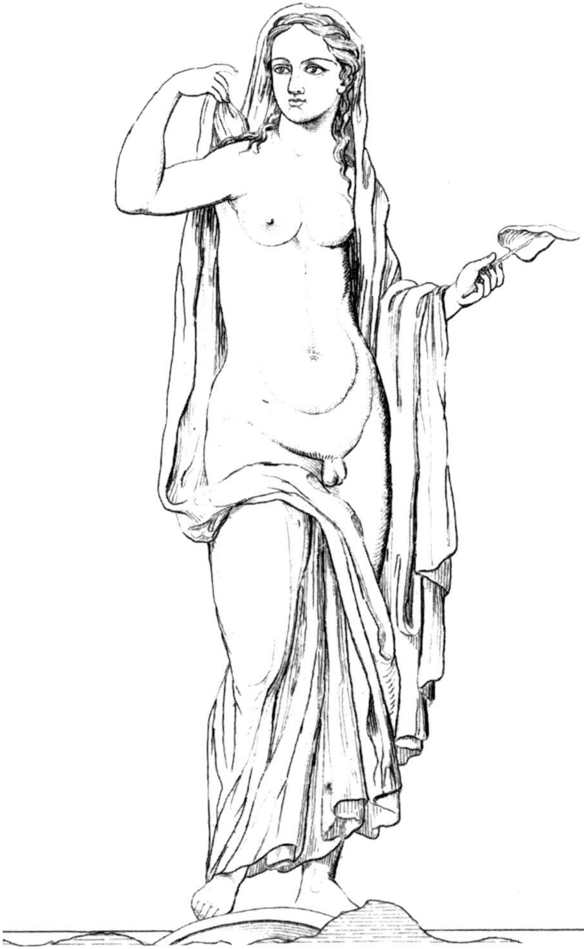

dition. The sixteenth-century Rabbi Joseph Karo codified Talmudic law and allotted each man sexual duties according to his occupation. Gentlemen of leisure should perform their duty every night. Labourers are obliged to perform twice a week, unless they work in another city, then they are let off with just once a week. So too for donkey drivers. Sailors, for obvious reasons, only once every six months. (So much for one in every port.)

In these circumstances men have no need to trouble their amorous heads; they know when and with whom (as the Talmud only sanctifies sex within marriage) they will be satisfied. And remember they are doing it

---

H. Roux, French (active 1840s).

Hermaphrodite. From the *Musée Secret.*

This "chick with a dick" was once a statue in Pompeii, which presumably is why that city incurred the wrath of the gods.

---

for God. It is written that Jewish men are known to be good lovers, for all they have to do is believe. Do they experience fewer sexual hang-ups because they have sex written into their faith? Woody Allen makes a conclusive case to the contrary in his films, but, perhaps between his own sheets, alone with his former adoptive daughter, he stumps up every time.

What then is the answer? Finding a way to make sex a part of our daily routine could help. In the ancient Chinese manual *Goddess of the Shell*, numerous ailments are treated with different sexual positions. For inner calm, a male should give 27 strokes of love to his supine partner, whilst kneeling

---

Louis André Berthommé-Saint-André, French (1905–77). Illustration from *Gamiani*.

Oh lucky man! Serviced from tip to toe, and his most relevant part in between. Should attention flag there is even an obliging nipple to give him a toe-job.

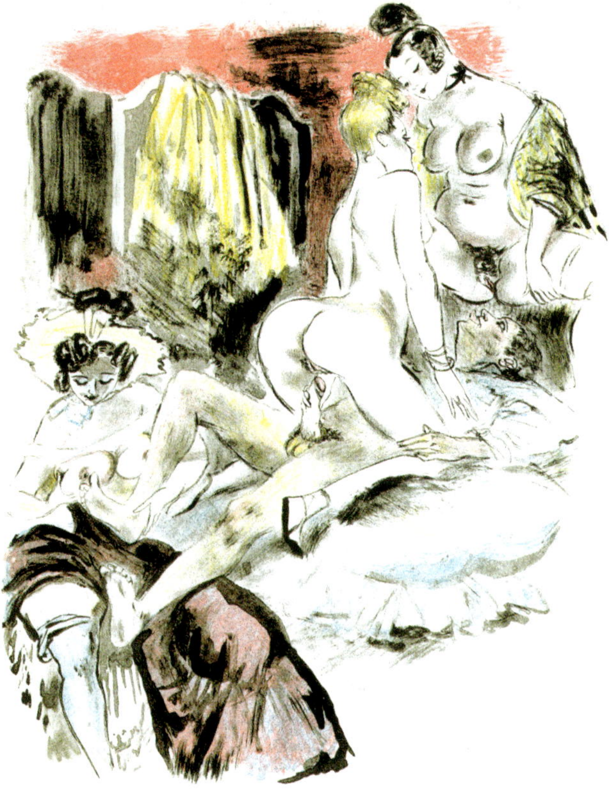

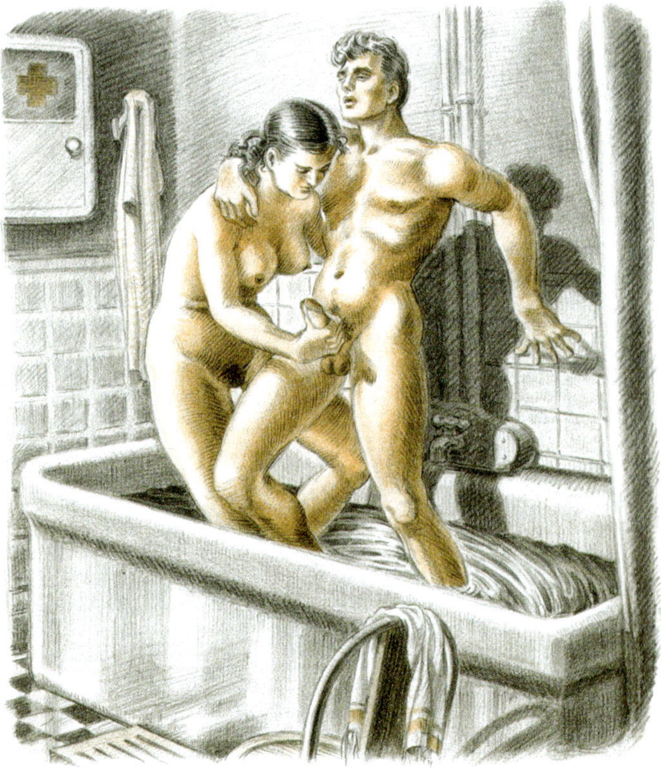

Anon., French (ca.1950).

Illustration from *Clayton's College.*

This buxom example of modern American collegiate loveliness is clearly majoring in practical anatomy and physical education.

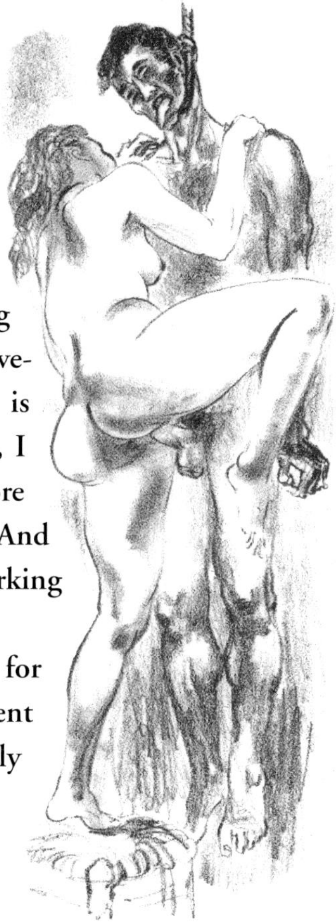

between her thighs. To be taken three times a day for twenty days.

If a man needs to improve his bone marrow, he must give 72 strokes, eight times daily, for as long as it takes to see an improvement. As bone marrow is tricky to monitor at home, I suspect the patient is far more likely to die of exhaustion. And may God rest his hard working little soul.

The important aspect for me, though, is that ancient Chinese culture implicitly understood sex to be a major aspect of all life, in a way that is barely understood in Occidental cultures. How can we expect the Western willy to stand up for itself in the face of such ignorance?

Finally, your cock is a muscle, and we all know how beneficial going to the gym is. Doctors and laymen alike believe the axiom: "Use it or lose it". This makes good sense, and is borne out by practice. I have personal experience of how effective

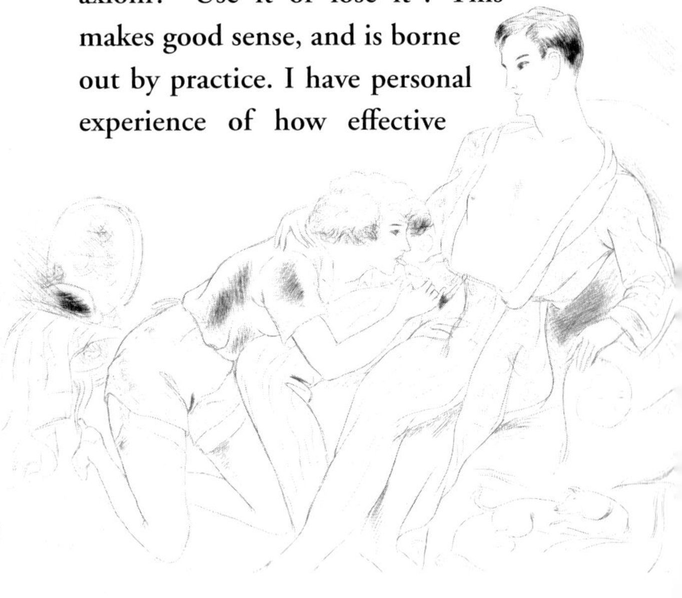

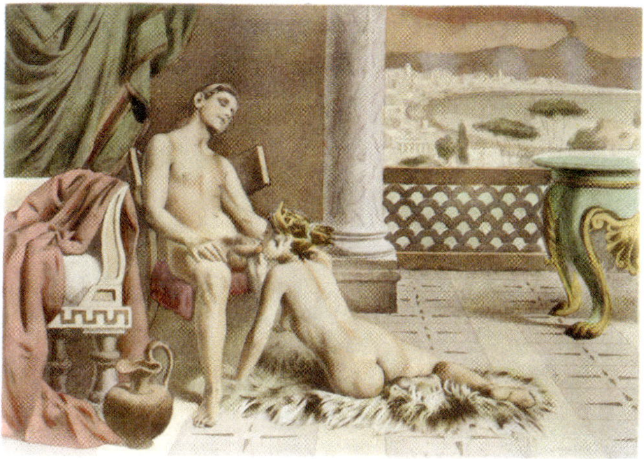

Above: Paul Avril, French (1849–1928).

Atalanta and Meleagro. From *De Figuris Veneris.*

In the background Vesuvius looks as if it is just about to blow, like Meleagro in the foreground. Atalanta is obviously a virtuoso player on the pink oboe.

Left: Léon Courbouleix, French (active 1930s).

Entre ses lèvres. Illustration from *Pour toi, pour moi*

"She catches his prick between her red lips, licking the glans and giving him a lingering suck while her hand gropes the balls of her beloved little fellow, who immediately perks up."

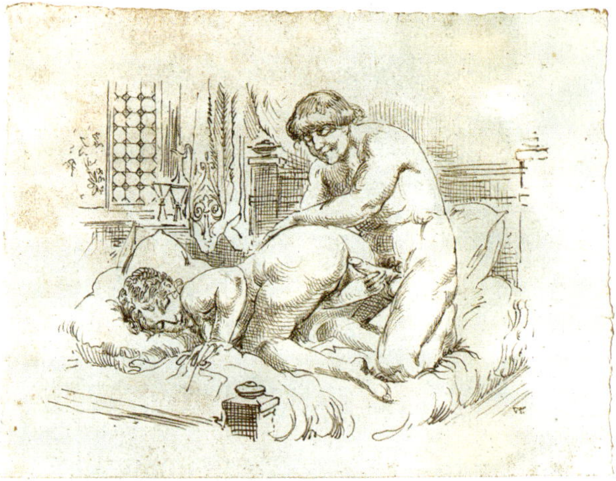

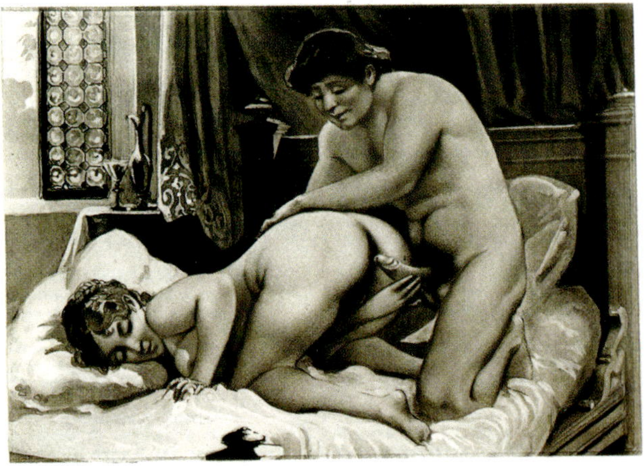

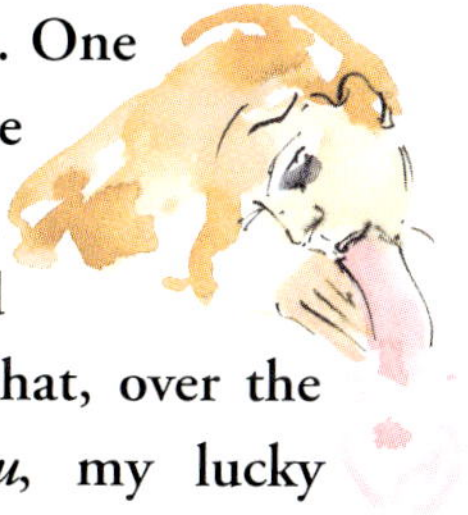

non-stop shagging can be. One of my ex-lovers and I were absolutely mad for each other, and at it day and night. We both noticed that, over the time of this *amour fou*, my lucky friend's todger became firmer and wider. Sadly, grand passions like this are difficult to maintain, as they preclude involvement with the real world, and so we inevitably ground to a halt. But when I recall our prodigious exploits, I do so hate to think of all that muscle turning to fat. However the

---

Opposite, above: French School (ca.1907).

Illustration from *Les Sonnets Luxurieux de L'Aretin.*

An illustration to Aretino's scandalous poem sequence, and supposed "antique" model for the picture below. The wickedly grinning *signorina* here is giving her chap an appreciative rub while guiding him to his haven.

Opposite, below: The lady's grin is a little less wicked, the fellow's weapon is a shade smaller. But her hand is no less grasping.

moral remains and if I may use the words of the immortal Homer Simpson: "It's good for what ails ya".

Of course, it is sometimes difficult for women to imagine the torments an insecure and sensitive chap may go through. Tending, as we do, to have idealised views of what a treat it must be to have a lovely lump o' love at your disposal. Stephen Berkoff, in *East*, gives Sylv this classic line:

> ...that super unworrisome flesh that toys between your thighs, that we must genuflect and kneel to, that we are beaten across the skull with... Nay, not fair that those pricks get all the fun.

Louis André Berthommé-Saint-André, French (1905–77).

La Bergère. From *Pybrac.*

This buxom shepherdess rides her man's saddle in the lush Normandy pastures. The cows for their part look unmoved. But then, perhaps they have the *vache folle* malaise.

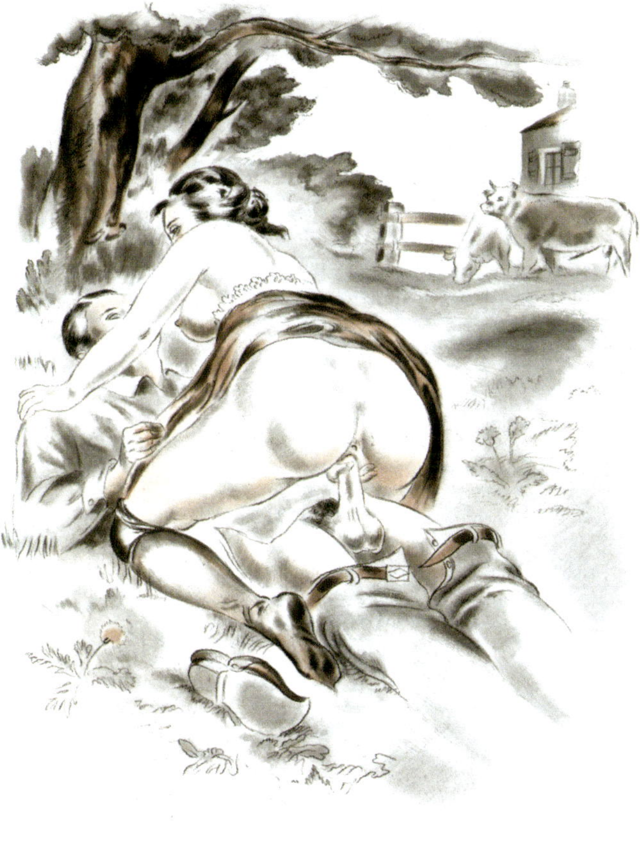

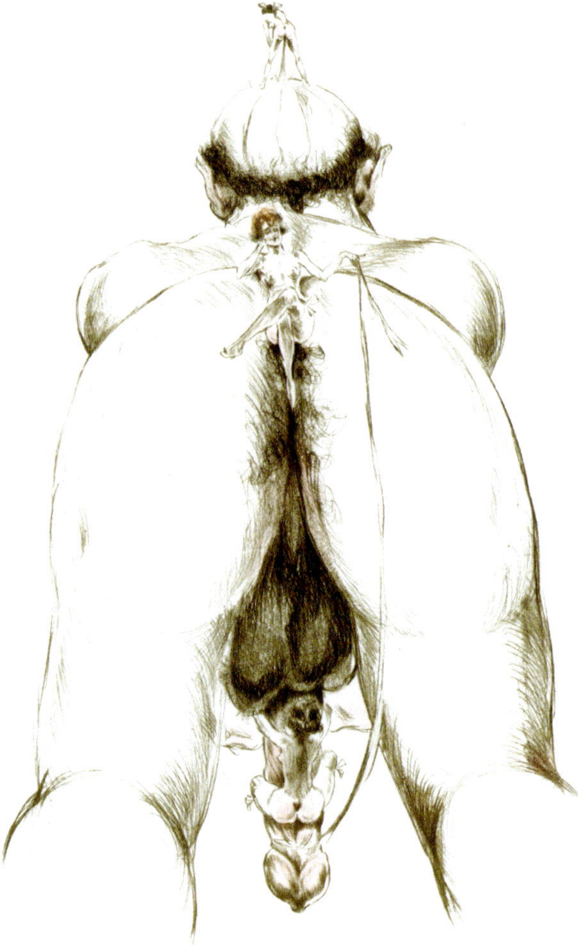

So you must forgive us, if we girls seem unsympathetic at times. It's simply that we are incredulous. How can having a penis *possibly* be a problem?

OVEREXPOSURE

FAR from being taken for granted, the sight of a dick is still a delight. This may be due to the double-edged sword of censorship. Ol' One Eye has still managed to retain a degree of mystique, despite doing the same routine for centuries. We are kept permanently wanting more.

"Pipifax", German (ca.1920).

The Swing. From *Erotische Grotesken.*

This mighty giant's bald head gets a good anointing from his pocket Venus, while two other diminutive sporting girls enjoy a game of slides in the crevice of his buttocks and swinging down his long pole.

It may sound as though I am in favour of censorship, but I am in trying to make the best of the ridiculous set of restrictions in this country. The long tradition of believing sex to be an evil or a weakness was instrumental in creating pornography. For what you are forbidden to do to your lover, you can watch hell-bound deviants do to one another. And from this came censorship; the jealous zealots trying to stop the party.

In biology classes we are shown flaccid members, and then teased by being told that this shaft becomes engorged and

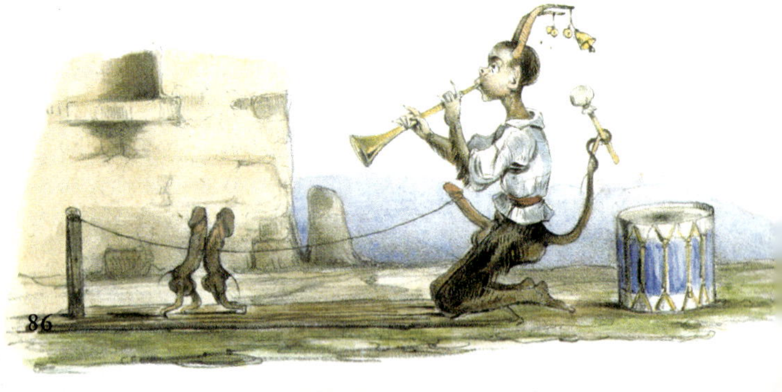

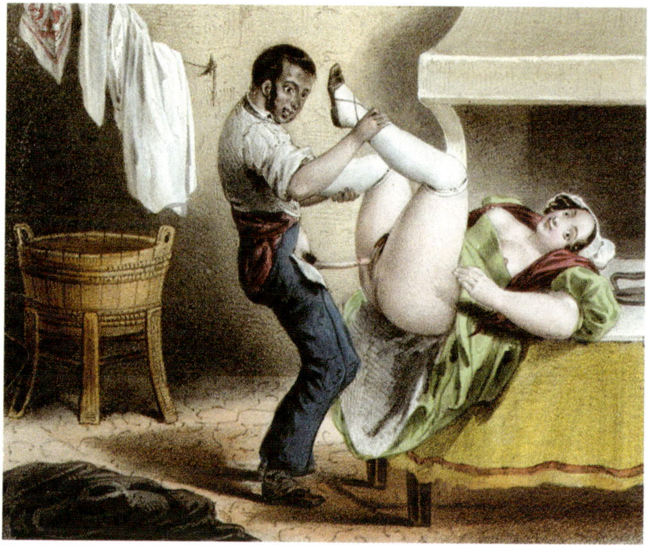

French School (ca.1830)

Ante Bellum.

Quel fusil! Every Southern Belle's fantasy come true. Harriet Beecher Stowe would not have been amused.

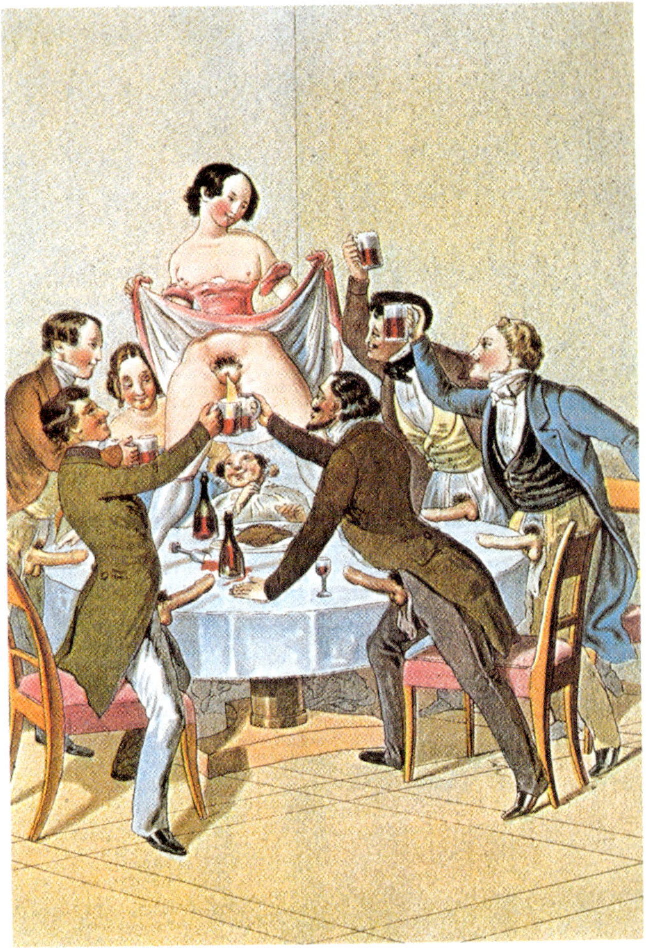

grows. But imagination will always outstrip mere fact. And so ill-informed girls in ankle socks run screaming in horror from the science labs. In their adolescent dreams they are chased through darkened corridors, pursued by huge, lumbering one-eyed monsters, craving virgin blood.

What possible harm is there in showing an erect penis? Half the population has their own, to peruse at their leisure, and the other half can safely expect to encounter one at some stage. I must confess that in fallow seasons I sometimes wonder if I'll ever get lucky again, but my mother taught me always to expect the unexpected. And wear clean underwear, in case it's a runaway bus.

Peter Fendi, Austrian (1796–1842).

The Toast.

Five clubbable young bucks recharge their glasses at the fount of all goodness. And then whack their payment out on the table.

AN END IN ITSELF

MOST contradictory and provocative of organs. You can be vulnerable, sensitive, and coy. Then like a coiled serpent you spring to life transforming into an aggressive, solid shaft, a life force, an item to be reckoned with.

This is why I adore you so. You pretend to ignore me, to feed my insecurity I'm sure, but always with one eye on me. You demurely turn your head whilst demanding my kisses; still watching. You fascinate me. Almost imperceptibly you move, so I bite you, only lightly. You seem to decide I'll put up a good fight, so you begin your gradual ascent.

P. F. Hugues d'Hancarville, French (active 1780s).

From *Monumens du Culte Secret des Dames Romaines.*

This little fellow is taking his first faltering steps towards greater things. But on the legs of a *chicken*?

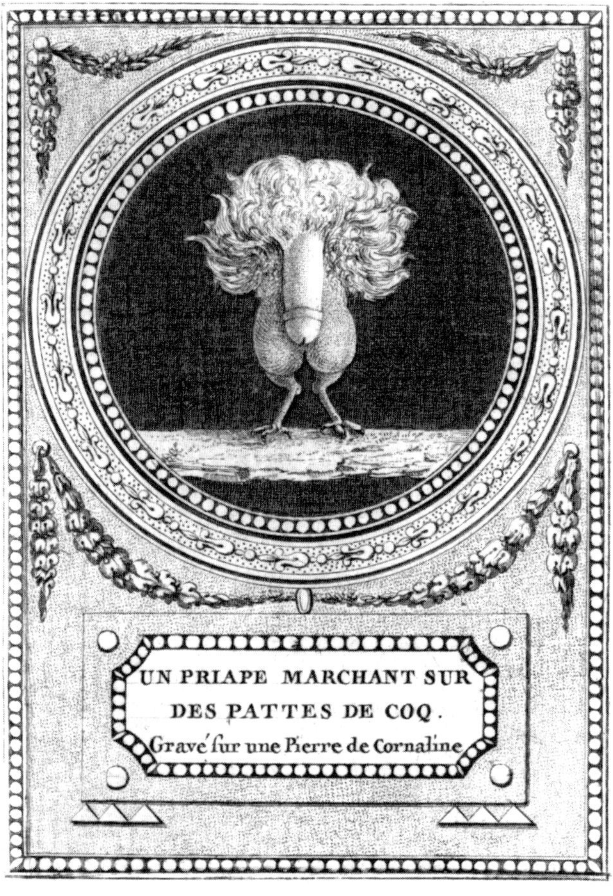
UN PRIAPE MARCHANT SUR
DES PATTES DE COQ.
Gravé sur une Pierre de Cornaline

This is most appealing. I, the wily snake charmer, breathing life into my enigmatic adversary, preparing my competitor for battle. It's just so damned exciting. Don't get me wrong, I like you almost as much in repose. I delight in the silky looseness of your flesh, the seemingly innocent appearance of you as you bury yourself within yourself. Simply exquisite. I, like you, am rivetted. Captivated by our joint

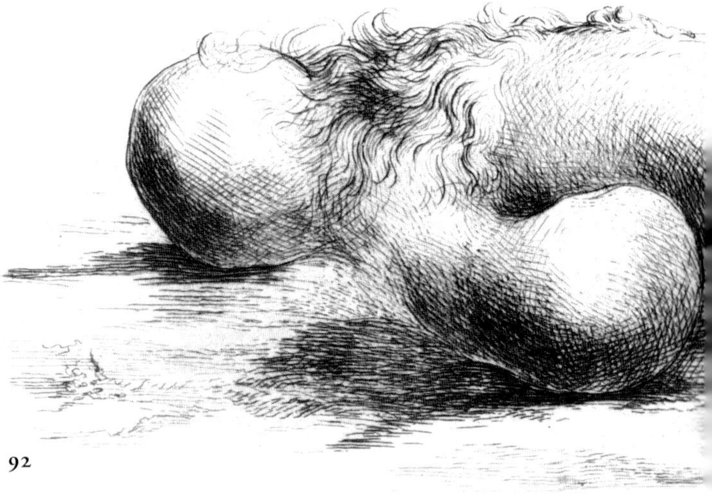

mission, the allure of the unknown, for as any experienced warrior knows: no two missions are alike.

If I worship you, it is because you give me so much pleasure and ask so little in return. Just a little water and a place to rest your head. It is your master who complicates our relations. Were it not for him, we would enjoy carefree times. Is it any wonder then that so many images of phallic worship in this book involve a detached member?

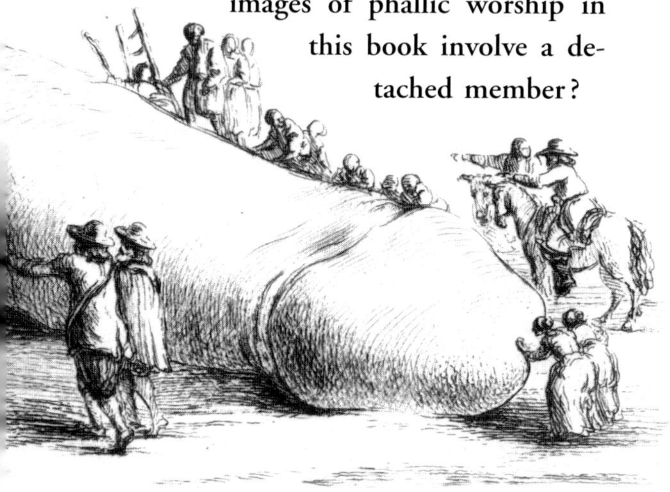

Vignettes and in-text illustrations:

Previous Spread: Vivant Dominique, Baron Denon, French (1747–1842).

The Beached Phallus. From *Œuvres Priapiques.*

Denon's 18th century version of a Dutch 17th century print, *The Beached Whale.* If, as the myth would have it, an owner's nose is as big as his penis, then one sneeze and its "goodbye Naples".

"Pipifax", German (ca.1920).

Variety Show. From *Erotische Grotesken.*

A charming member of the *corps de ballet* has remembered to wear her tutu, but alas has forgotten her leotard, for this command performance.

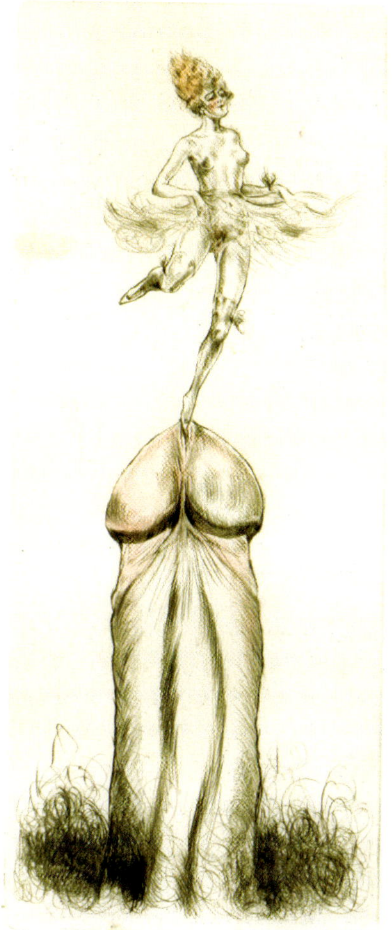

Variété I/82. Pipifax

Our Freephone orderline is 0800 026 25 24
You can email us at *eros@eroticprints.org*
Or visit us on the Internet at
www.eroticprints.org

This edition copyright © 1999 MacHo Ltd.

First published in 1999 by THE *Erotic* Print Society
Reprinted September 2002

Printed and bound in Spain by Bookprint, S.L., Barcelona

Designed at Cypher
12 ST MARTIN'S COURT ULLSWATER ROAD SE27

ISBN: 1-898998-55-8

No part of this publication may be reproduced by any means without the express written permission of the publishers. The moral right of the author and all the illus-trators included in this publication have been asserted.